STAIRS FOR BREAKFAST

An inspiring memoir by a man with
Cerebral Palsy who doesn't let anything
stand in his way

By
Patrick Souiljaert

ISBN-13: 978-1986090544
ISBN-10: 198609054X

This book has been printed by
CPI Group (UK) Ltd, Croydon, CR0 4YY
www.cpi-print.co.uk

Praise For Stairs For Breakfast

"When someone tells me they can't do something I tell them Patrick's story and share his ability to overcome whatever is put in front of him. He is an inspiration."

Glenn Armstrong,
www.glennarmstrong.com

"Patrick consulted me while writing this book. This book is a must for anyone. It's honest, funny and inspirational. It humbles me just thinking about the effort it must have taken."

Paul Ribbons,
www.paulribbons.com

"An enormous achievement. Do yourself a favour. Add it to your reading wish list – and those of your friends"

Roy Stannard

Contents

Foreword

Stairs for Breakfast by Patrick Souiljaert is a raw testament to the fact that courage comes in all sorts of shapes and sizes and that human endeavour can overcome just about any obstacle. It is the first-hand account of someone who was born with Cerebral Palsy and a first rate brain and the connections that have had to be made throughout his life to convince others of his worth.

Displaying an amazing recall with a photographic memory for the exact detail of conversations and experiences, Patrick takes us through every emotional pothole in his life without any attempt to finesse the detail or spare the feelings of those who made the mistake of treating him as any less of a human being because of his condition.

The title of the book comes from the regular encounters that Patrick has had with climbing stairs – something that lesser determined individuals would have found ways of bypassing. The names of most people in the book have been changed to protect sensibilities.

As the book progresses from childhood to teenage years, schooldays and on to his working life it is clear that the journey has become steeper and more treacherous as life has moved on. Some of the routine prejudice and condescension experienced beggars belief. All of it is recorded forensically.

The experience is akin to being given access to someone's personal diaries. The pain and occasionally the joy runs like blood off the page. However, his quick wit and natural humour also suffuses the book. This is someone who can see the funny side and this leaps off the page.

The underlying theme of the book is Patrick's search for a soul mate – someone who accepts him for who he is – and loves him for it. As writing this book is part of that journey and exposes large bruised chunks of that soul, I suspect that the person he is seeking is probably going to read it.

An enormous achievement. Do yourself a favour. Add it to your reading wish list – and those of your friends.

Roy Stannard
Friend

Introduction

Everybody creates their own reality (and perception): for example, I could think that my life is too difficult, and I could decide to give up and go and live in a residential home for disabled people. Instead I have always thought, *I can do anything I want to in life.*

Everybody has the power to choose how they live in life. Ultimately, it comes down to the thoughts you have about yourself (and about other people) and the decisions you make.

You can overcome and achieve anything you want in life. All you need is enough self-belief and desire.

I've always liked challenging myself by doing the impossible – things which *I know* I can do but which some people tell me I won't be able to do. *Stairs For Breakfast* is giving me a platform as a public speaker. I love speaking about overcoming adversity and inspiring people to achieve whatever you want to do.

Going into property investment and leaving my £30K IT job is the best decision I've made so far in life. I've learnt so much about people and success over the last five years. It has led me to realise what my purpose is in life: to help and inspire people – and to reach my full potential.

My main motivation for writing a book on overcoming adversity is because I want to inspire people and I would like to make a difference in the world.

Although everything in this book is the absolute truth. I deeply love my mum and wish her no ill will. My hope for Mum is for her to be happy and at peace with herself and with my aunt and uncle

I thought about my autobiography for two-and-a-half years, before I started to write it. Once I began it, it took me fifteen months to type it (with my left index finger). Upon completion, Stephanie Hale (my publishing adviser) said to me "216,000 words is too long for one book, I suggest splitting it into two books." The sequel is planned for publication in the next year or two.

Many people in the property investment community have inspired me and have become friends. I would especially like to thank Glenn Armstrong and Paul Ribbons. Individually, they have taught, helped and inspired me so much. The thing which makes me feel very humble is, they both really want me to succeed.

When I finished writing my autobiography Paul and Glenn advised me "To cover the cost of publishing *Stairs For Breakfast*, create a webpage for people to pre-order the book." So I did – and that is what has happened. Thank you Juswant & Sylvia Rai (Berkshire Property Meet) and John Cox (Bucks Property Meet) for promoting my book.

I would also like to thank Alex Wade for his legal advice and Jon Santa Cruz for the front cover photo.

Recently, I did a book talk in front of twenty people. I was feeling slightly nervous beforehand, but once I started, I was in my element! I had considered creating a Powerpoint presentation and decided not to.

My 'off the top of my head' talk was excellent. I spoke for an hour-and-a-quarter and interacted well with the audience. People asked lots of questions and I loved it! The feedback afterwards was very good.

The thought of speaking in front of hundreds of people scares me but I know I can do it. It's just a matter of feeling the fear and doing it anyway!

I am proud of *Stairs For Breakfast* and hope you enjoy it.

Chapter 1

I was due to be born on 2nd December 1973. But there were complications. A couple of weeks beforehand, my mum wasn't feeling well, so she went to the hospital to get checked over. Upon being examined, she was told, "There's a problem. You've got extremely high blood pressure and we need to induce the birth immediately."

I entered the world on 21st November 1973 at Masons Hill Maternity Hospital in Bromley, Kent, the only time I've arrived early for something in my life!

The umbilical cord had become twisted and was wrapped around my neck, preventing me from breathing for the first four minutes of my life. After which point I gave out a little cough and started to breathe normally.

The midwife said to my mum, "Your son is fine but he might have some learning difficulties."

It was only when I was nine months old – when my parents realised I had difficulty sitting up properly – that I was diagnosed with Cerebral Palsy (CP).

CP is a result of damage to the brain, due to oxygen starvation at birth.

* * * *

Hi, my name is Patrick Souiljaert and this is my life (so far). I have overcome and achieved some amazing things. My mindset and determination are my greatest assets. However, the overriding factor to my success is that I have never thought of, nor seen myself as being disabled. I know what I can accomplish and I have never let anything, or anyone, get in my way. I've got a 'do or die' attitude to life.

I am going to take you on a journey through my life. From my earliest memory to where I am today. I have been through some dark and difficult times. But don't worry, I have overcome them all. I like setting myself 'impossible' goals; things that other people see as impossible but I know I can do. And I achieve every goal I set myself. I've always believed that I will achieve something extraordinary in life.

I hope you enjoy reading my book.

* * * *

First of all, a bit of housekeeping! The question I get asked the most is, "How do you pronounce your surname?" (sue-lee-art) followed by, "Where does it come from?" (Belgium).

My dad was born and raised in Antwerp. My mum was born and grew up in East London. They met in Dar es Salaam (East Africa) in the 1960s – where my dad was working and my mum was on holiday.

My dad likes to recount stories of the few years he spent in the navy when he was young. However, he spent most of his working life in a corporate job working for International Metal Services (IMS). Every few years he would get a promotion to become the director of one IMS' larger sites. This often involved moving to another country.

I have one sister, Clare, who is twenty months older than me.

* * * *

I reckon I have a recollection of the few minutes just after I was born. I can remember bright lights (like in an operating theatre), being wrapped in a white blanket and then being placed in a see-through container, which had a lid on it (that I once described as a breadbin!) Who knows? Maybe being starved of oxygen made my brain really alert.

When I was about eight-years-old, I told my mum about my recollection of the few minutes after I was born. She replied, "Nah, you must have dreamt it." But she then said that the white blanket and being placed in an incubator sounded about right.

Before moving to Belgium in 1976, Dad worked in London and we lived in Bromley. I must have been about two when I developed a fascination with worms! I used to crawl around the back garden and knew there was a part of it where there were worms. I would pick one up, with my left hand, have a close look at it, hold the other end of the worm with my right hand – and then pull it apart. I would then put the worm back on the ground and watch in fascination as the two halves wiggled around and marvel at the fact that they were still alive. I would then pick one of the halves up again and pull it apart. It was a disgusting habit and my first lesson in multiplication!

Dad got promoted to run an IMS subsidiary near Liege. Neither football nor geography has ever been my strong point but I think the only thing Liege is known for is having a reasonably well-known football team – Standard Liege.

We lived in a rented house in a suburb of Liege called Embourg. The house was situated down a long, steep drive, in a slightly forested area. There was one house next door and Luke who lived there (with his family) was a dentist and also owned the house we lived in.

Our house had an open plan living room, with French doors to the back garden at one end and stairs at the other. There were two sets of stairs – four or five steps, leading down to the front door and the toilet, and a flight of wide wooden steps up to the first floor. Upstairs there were three bedrooms and the bathroom.

The stairs up to the first floor had no backs to them. This made it easy for me to crawl up them and I grabbed hold of each wooden step, with my left hand, as I went up them. At first, I did the same thing in reverse, going down the stairs; I went down them backwards, again holding on to each step with my left hand. It wasn't long before my confidence grew and I was gliding down the stairs, head first, on my tummy!

There was another bedroom on the ground floor at the front of the house, which, oddly, was only accessible from the outside of the property. This is where my grandparents used to sleep when they came to visit. Next to this bedroom was a double garage.

The back garden had a fairly large round swimming pool in it. We had a cat called Peter. He was white with big ginger spots.

I used to crawl everywhere – up and down the stairs and in the front and back garden. There was nowhere I couldn't get to.

I'm left handed and the left side of my body has always been stronger (less affected by my CP) than my right side. I used to crawl with my right hand closed, putting the back of my hand on the floor. This caused my right knuckles to become very hard and they used to develop cracks and bleed. My parents encouraged me to crawl with my right hand flat – as I did with my left hand.

Another thing I used to do was dribble all of the time. I used to be a real dribbler (and I am not referring to playing basketball). Sometimes I dribbled so much it made my chin red and sore. Mum was always telling me, "Stop dribbling", especially when we went out somewhere, but it had little effect on me.

I find it strange talking about me crawling around and dribbling everywhere because it was so long ago.

When we went out I used a buggy. If we weren't going very far one of my parents (usually Mum) would carry me, with my feet around their waist. Clare was able to carry me by the time she was ten (and she could still carry me up until I got to about twenty-three).

A key to my success in life has been my family because they have never treated me as if I am disabled. My parents (Mum slightly more so than Dad) always encouraged me to do things for myself and to be independent.

On the upstairs landing of our house, overlooking the living room, we had a large fish tank which had several big and colourful tropical fish in it.

When I was about four, I had a small fish tank containing a goldfish in my bedroom. The rectangular tank was on a shelf at the head of my bed. I used to watch the fish when I went to bed. One night, while I was feeling warm and cosy under my duvet, I suddenly felt sorry for my goldfish; there I was in my warm bed and there was the fish in cold water. *It must be cold*, I thought. So I put my hand in the tank, scooped out the fish and laid it on the right side of my pillow, pulling up my duvet over the fish to keep it warm! I remember the fish flapping around for a bit before it went to sleep. When I woke up in the morning I learned a lesson about fish!

My family knew I was intelligent before I started to speak at the age of four. One of the very first words I said was "Fire!"

It's a mystery to me why I started talking at a relatively late age. Perhaps my CP may have caused me to be a bit shy.

Dad had a cream-coloured three door Range Rover. Weirdly it had two fuel tanks – a petrol one and a diesel one. There was a switch down by the gear sticks to determine which fuel you wanted to use before starting the engine.

I've always enjoyed listening to the radio and music – and like a multitude of songs from the 1950s through to today. 'Fire' by The Pointer Sisters isn't one of my favourite songs but it's a poignant one.

My fifth birthday will always be a happy memory. When I woke up that morning there was something very big in the corner of my room, covered up with a white sheet. I had no idea what it could be. I remember the few seconds of anticipation I felt before discovering what it was. I had never got out of bed or crawled somewhere so fast!

As I pulled the white sheet off my birthday present, my anticipation turned into joy and excitement. It was a red battery-operated motorbike.

Up until that point, the only way I had of getting around was by crawling everywhere. The motorbike gave me a new lease of life.

Initially, I rode it around the lounge and kept crashing into things (furniture, walls and people!). All I wanted to do was to ride it at full speed! Like standard motorbikes, the acceleration was on the right handle. I very quickly grasped how to twist the accelerator to make the motorbike go faster. But I was reluctant to let go of the accelerator and wasn't very good at stopping! I liked the sensation of speed!

In the beginning, I rode the motorbike at full speed down the stairs, leading to the front door! I felt balanced holding onto the bike with both hands. The thought of letting go with my right hand, and losing my balance, scared me more than riding the motorbike down the stairs. After doing so on two or three occasions, each time falling off and hurting myself, I learnt to let go of the accelerator.

It taught me to have more control of my right hand. It wasn't long before I was riding my bike slowly and in full control. Also, I quickly learnt how to get myself on and off of it. I was soon riding my motorbike in the front and back garden.

My parents were friends with an English family who lived near us called Sue and Tony Meadows, who had two kids named Jane and Ian. Clare and I were friends with Jane and Ian. Jane was a year older than me (Ian was three years older than I was). I quite liked Jane because she always talked to me which was kind. We were also friends with two American families who lived in Embourg.

I started school at the age of five and attended a French-speaking school for the disabled in the centre of Liege. A taxi (a black saloon Mercedes – all taxis in Liege at the time were black – and most of them were Mercedes), picked me up and took me home every day. The school run entailed picking other people up on the way. My journey to and from school took forty-five minutes.

Clare went to the local school, five minutes away. I felt it was unfair that I had to leave home for school before Clare did and get home after her. However, there was nothing I could do about it, so I accepted it.

At school I got myself around in a manual wheelchair. My early memories of school in Belgium include the way my teacher first taught my class to read and write (in French – obviously).

The teacher did so using a series of little square cards. On each card was a picture of a person, an action or an object. We had to put several cards together to form a sentence.

For instance; a picture of a boy, followed by a picture of a leg and foot doing a kicking action, followed by a picture of a ball, apparently spells (according to Google) 'Le garçon est à botter le ballon' (the boy is kicking the ball).

I've always thought this was a strange way of teaching kids to read and write because it didn't teach me to read or to write in French (or in English, nor in any other language for that matter). Also, was my teacher making fun of us small children in wheelchairs? Playing football has never been my forté.

My favourite subject at school was maths and anything involving numbers. I have always had an excellent memory when it comes to remembering numbers. The same cannot be said with me and names however!

Back at home, it became obvious from an early age that Dad was the one who went out to work, whilst Mum was primarily the one who looked after Clare and me. I don't remember Dad being around much during the week as he left the house for work before Clare and I left to go to school in the mornings. He also played squash once or twice a week in the evening. During the week Dad was focussed on his work. At the weekends he was more relaxed.

Clare and I got on well. Like any young siblings we would sometimes fight but she would always help me if I needed it.

For Mum, Clare and I, English is our primary language. I must have been five when Clare and I started to speak French with Dad. It was easy learning to speak French at that age. I don't recall having any difficulty understanding things at school. Clare and I have spoken French with Dad ever since. Mum always encouraged me to do as much as possible and to be independent, whereas Dad sometimes held me back. When I was small, he tended to involve, and show things to, Clare more than me.

One example was when he was showing Clare how the hifi in the lounge worked. I asked, "Can I have a go...?"

I remember Dad saying to me, "Tu veux toujours toucher a tout," (You always want to touch everything). And, "Ne touche pas ca, tu vas le casser." (Don't touch that, you are going to break it.)

I resented this because I felt Dad was being unfair. I couldn't understand why Clare had the freedom to touch the stereo and I didn't. Another difficulty was that I sometimes found it hard to express myself and how I was feeling.

I have always been interested in how things work (especially electrical things and anything related to music). I've always had the opinion that the best way of learning is by doing. Which is why, today, I am good at using computers. I've never been afraid of trying to do something new on my computer – and I have never broken it!

It was unusual for Dad to go to his office at the weekend. However, I did go with him a couple of times. I particularly remember one occasion, when he needed to do something, briefly.

His office was in a rectangular building and the entrance was in the centre at the front, through a set of double doors. Dad carried me as he unlocked one of the doors and we went in. To the left were some small offices, with Dad's being at the far end. To the right was an open-plan office.

There was nobody else in the building so Dad let me crawl around, while he went into his office to do whatever he had to do. I crawled up the corridor into the open-plan office. There were several rows of desks to the right and to the left. As I crawled up the centre of the room, looking at all of the desks and chairs, I noticed that each desk had a phone on it, some pens and small square blocks of paper pads with 'IMS' printed on the side of them (I recognised the blocks of paper pads because we had some at home). It was at that moment that I thought, *I am going to work in an office like this one day.*

Before I started to speak at the age of four, I knew I was bright because I understood everything that went on around me. My mind has always been very active and I knew that one day I would achieve great things in life.

Throughout Dad's career at IMS he had a company car. While living in Belgium he either had a BMW or a Mercedes.

One weekend, when Dad had a BMW, the four of us were on our way home from visiting my grandparents in Antwerp, when we had a crash. We were on the motorway when one of the BMW's tyres burst. It caused the car to spin around a couple of times and hit the barrier on the hard shoulder. Dad managed to keep control of the car and when it came to a stop we were facing in the right direction! Fortunately, we didn't collide with any other vehicles and none of us were hurt. Dad changed the tyre and drove home. When we arrived home, I remember seeing how badly damaged the back of the car was. Part of the rear bumper had disintegrated and all of the lights were smashed. I realised how lucky we were not to have been injured.

We went to see my paternal grandparents about once a month. They lived on the third floor of a modern apartment block in Antwerp. The ground floor communal area, leading up to the stairs and lift, had marble walls and floor and was very echoey. My grandparents weren't rich but they were comfortable (they were both teachers and my Granny later became a headmistress). Their apartment had three bedrooms and a nice soft carpet for me to crawl on! They spoke Flemish, French and a bit of English, but I only remember speaking with them in French.

My Granny enjoyed cooking and, most of the time, made nice meals when we went to see them. She always made the same starter, as it was Clare's favourite. 'Tomates crevettes' – shrimps mixed with mayonnaise and served in a large hollowed- out, uncooked tomato. I quite liked it as well.

However, on one occasion, she cooked 'lapin aux pruneaux' (rabbit with prunes). I'm not sure about Mum and Dad, but it didn't go down well with Clare and me! I will always remember my Granny for the delicious waffles she made. She made a ton of them whenever we went to visit. And we would take home two or three large containers, filled with fresh waffles.

After lunch every day Grandpa went for an hour's nap but, when we were there, he always liked to have a mug of tea with Clare and me first. Drinking tea was something we only did with Grandpa because at home Clare and I drank coffee.

Grandpa had a cine-camera and had footage of Clare and I when we were extremely young. I also remember Grandpa having a Betamax video recorder.

In a field near where my grandparents lived was a horse (I don't recall whose horse it was). We used to go and feed it carrots and sugar lumps. Although I held my hand flat in doing so, I was always scared the horse was going to bite my hand (it never did)! Dad and Clare have always been into horses.

My maternal grandparents, on the other hand, lived in a two-bed council maisonette in Hackney, in the rough East End of London. And they relied on their state pension to get by. We went to see them during the school holidays. My Nan was one of the nicest people you could ever meet. She would do anything for anybody. However, my Grandad wasn't a very pleasant man. He was deaf as a post (which didn't help matters). He often shouted at my Nan, "Sally – come and help me..." He also went around coughing and farting a lot!

Grandad wasn't a very generous man either. Every Christmas, he would take some money out of his pocket and give Clare and I (and my three cousins) £1 each. I'm sure once, as he gave me the £1 he said, "Spend it wisely..."

The toilet in Nan and Grandad's flat was up a long flight of stairs. When I was extremely young, Nan had a potty for me to wee into – in the lounge!

Nan used to take Clare and me to her bingo club. The first time we went I won a box of tea! After that Clare said I was a lucky person. Every time we went again Clare said that I would win something. Sometimes I did!

Nan also used to take Clare and me to the West End. She would say, "We're going up the West End to feed the pigeons." (At Trafalgar Square.)

Wherever Nan took us in London we always got the number 38 bus back to Hackney. Being a bit grumpy, Grandad never came with us. He liked going down the betting shop and having a small bet on the horses.

To make us laugh Nan often did handstands up against the upstairs wall. She was still doing handstands at seventy-eight years old!

During the holidays we also saw my aunt and uncle (Mum's sister and brother-in-law) and my three cousins. We would either see them at Nan and Grandad's or go to their house in Shoreham-by-Sea.

One Christmas we were all at Nan and Grandad's – where all five of us kids slept in the same bedroom. When we woke up on Christmas day, Damian (my eldest cousin, who's eight years older than me), convinced us that he had woken up in the middle of the night and seen Father Christmas outside the window!

It was while we were staying at Nan and Grandad's (when I was five or six) that Mum said me, "When you're older they will have invented a computer chip and implanted it into your brain to help you walk and talk properly." I had my doubts and implanting a computer chip in my brain sounded a bit dangerous to me.

In the summer of 1979 we (Mum, Dad, Clare and I) went on holiday to Greece. I enjoyed swimming in the outdoor pool with my armbands on and holding my head under the water, I particularly liked sitting on the side of the pool and diving into it. I was confident diving in and swimming with my armbands on. However, Mum wanted to get me swimming without armbands. So, she stood in the pool near to where I dived in and made sure I resurfaced! It was a bit scary at first but after doing it a few times my confidence grew.

I liked diving in and touching the bottom of the pool with my hand. This gave Mum an idea. When I was in the water, she threw a coin to the bottom of the pool and gave my back a little push. I then swam to the bottom and picked up the coin. After having done so a few times, Mum threw two coins to the bottom of the pool. Mum gave me a push, down I swam and picked up both coins. I got to picking three coins up at once. I laughed every time I resurfaced holding the coins. I enjoyed the challenge and having something to aim for, which I knew I could achieve. It also taught me to hold my breath for ages! I was like a little dolphin!

On holiday, for a few minutes after getting out of the swimming pool I got cramp in my legs (especially my right leg), but I didn't know what it was. I thought that water had somehow got into my legs! I kept saying, "My leg hurts. I've got water in it..."

After that holiday, we regularly went swimming at the weekends with Sue, Tony, Jane and Ian. There were two local swimming pools. One was at the Holiday Inn, where we sometimes ate afterwards. The other swimming pool had three diving boards of different heights – Clare and Jane liked jumping off of the highest one. Dad carried me up there and I tried it once. Rather them than me!

We didn't use the swimming pool in our garden *that* much because it wasn't heated. The water was only warm enough in the summer. Delphine, a girl who I went to school with (in the same taxi as me), came to swim in our pool with us a few times.

It got pretty cold during the winter in Belgium. I think we got more use out of our swimming pool then. The pool would ice over. The ice was so thick that friends would come over and we used the pool as an ice skating rink! I say 'we' but I just crawled around on the ice! It's not something I would advise people to do today. What can I say? It was the 1970s.

In winter, it often snowed heavily enough for people to put snow tyres or tyre chains on their cars. The long steep drive down to our house was sometimes tricky to negotiate. After my taxi driver nearly failed to get back up the drive one morning, he wouldn't attempt it again. He didn't even bother coming to pick me up to go to school once or twice. On another occasion he waited at the top of our drive and started beeping his horn to let us know he was there! While Mum was pushing me in my buggy, up the steep drive in the snow and ice, I said "Wouldn't it be better for me to stay at home today?" But she didn't agree!

My interest in music was evident from a young age. On my sixth birthday I received a little portable cassette player and an ABBA tape (I think it may have been the 'Arrival' album, the cassette tape had a yellow label on it). I took my presents to school on my birthday and played ABBA loudly in my classroom!

It was at about this time that we got a puppy – a Briard (a French sheep dog) – called Zebedee. Our cat, Peter, didn't appreciate Zebedee much. Zebedee always wanted to play with Peter (and sniff Peter's butt!). But, being more placid, Peter just wanted to be left alone.

One Sunday evening while he was still a puppy, Zebedee was chewing a bone (trying to get the marrow from the inside of it), when he started yelping. He had somehow got the bone completely wedged between his teeth.

With it being Sunday evening and no vet nearby, Dad carried Zebedee over to Luke's house (our next door neighbour dentist). Dad, Clare and Luke (not forgetting Zebedee), then drove to Luke's practice. Picture this scene – eight-year-old Clare sitting in the dentist's chair, holding Zebedee in her arms, Dad holding the dog's mouth open, while Luke used some of his instruments to extract the bone from between his teeth!

It became apparent that whenever I sat down, my left foot would often cross over onto my right foot. This was due to my abductors being extremely tight (abductors are the group of muscles on the inside of your upper legs). Therefore, in the summer of 1980 I had an operation to release and lengthen my abductor muscles.

I remember the moments leading up to the operation being frightening. I was wheeled on a bed, into the operating theatre and then transferred onto the operating table. There were three men in white coats around me. A few minutes went by before one of the guys approached me holding a big black rubber mask. I laid there watching this big black mask as it got closer and closer to my face.

What the hell is it? I thought, as the mask was placed over my mouth and nose. I decided to put up a fight and pushed the mask off my face. It started a commotion. Every time they tried to put the mask on I used both of my hands to push it as far away as I could. Then two of the guys tried to hold my arms down on my chest but I kept fighting. They couldn't hold my arms well enough for the third person to hold the mask over my mouth and nose. Eventually, one of the men went and got someone else to help them. It took three guys to hold my arms down. The mask was only on my face for a few seconds before I lost consciousness.

Had someone told me beforehand that I was going to be gas masked, I probably wouldn't have been so scared. Come to think of it, I don't remember being asked if I minded having an operation either!

When I woke up after the operation I found myself in a hospital bed. I was covered in plaster of Paris and in a bit of discomfort. The plaster went from my ankles up to my hips, which prevented me from sitting up. Also, there was a piece of wood between my two lower legs – and moulded into plaster on each leg. This forced my legs wide apart and kept my abductors stretched. I wasn't expecting this to happen. I remember Mum being there and asking her, "What have they done to me?"

I spent six weeks of that summer lying down on a little foldable bed with wheels. I remember my family wheeling me around the lounge and in the back garden. Every so often they helped me to turn over from lying on my front, onto my back (and vice versa).

On the odd occasions when we went out somewhere I laid on the back seat of the car. Clare had the choice of having my head or my feet on her lap!

Dad taught me how to play draughts while I was in plaster, which I enjoyed.

Having the plaster taken off was a weird and scary experience as well. The guy who removed the plaster did so using an electric circular saw. He first removed the plaster from my right leg by sawing a line on the outside of my leg, from my ankle up to my hip. Then he moved onto the inside of right leg, sawing a line from my ankle up to my groin. The guy repeated the process on my left leg. At one point I thought I was going to have my manhood sawn off! Throughout the whole time of the sawing I kept being told, "Keep still... it won't hurt..."

The scary thing was the immense vibration the electric circular saw produced. Plaster of Paris isn't *that* thick. It felt like the guy was going saw into my legs. However, what was even more frightening was the heat generated by the electric saw. As I six-year-old boy, I thought my skin was going to be burned. This scared me more than the thought of having my leg sawn into.

When you've had your legs locked in plaster and been unable to move about for six weeks, having the plaster removed is one of the best feelings in the world! It also felt a bit strange because my legs felt a lot lighter (due to the loss of muscle tone).

I have had three operations on my legs and feet over the years. Having an operation and being in plaster for two to three months is a daunting, painful and annoying experience (due to being unable to get around much). However, I soon realised the long-term benefit of going through all of this, after coming out of the plaster and recovering from the operation. It means going through a short-term ordeal to having a life-changing experience. After seeing the improvement in my mobility and ability to walk I appreciated having the operations.

After recovering from my operation (in 1980) I started to have a lot more physiotherapy at school. I had physio for half an hour every morning. First of all, the physiotherapist would lay me on my back, on one of the six beds, in the massive physio room. She stretched my abductors and my hamstrings for about fifteen minutes. At the same time she got me to exercise my right hand. I laid both of my arms flat on the bed, alongside my body, and I had to keep opening and closing my right hand. When I stopped, every so often, the physio tapped me on my hand to tell me to keep on opening and closing it.

Next came my big, heavy, metal callipers – which came with their own pair of shoes (which I wore every day to school). The physio would put my callipers on me while I was still lying on the bed. The callipers went from my waist down to my shoes. There were two holes on each side of my shoes, for the callipers to plug into. The callipers contained a number of fastenings for each leg – a belt buckle strap around my waist, a Velcro strap around my upper legs, a knee pad with two small belt buckle fastenings, and a Velcro strap around my lower legs.

Once the physio had put my callipers on, she put me in my wheelchair and took me over to another part of the physio room, where there was a long wooden bench (the kind you find in a school gymnasium). She would then sit on the low bench whilst I stood in front of her (with my back to her). I then spent the next ten minutes standing up and balancing. The physio kept her hands close to my waist to ensure that I didn't fall over. And then I would take a couple of steps forward – but the callipers were far too heavy to walk in – they weren't meant for walking; they just held my legs completely straight. In taking a couple of steps, I resembled a penguin, hobbling from side to side!

A few feet in front of where I did my physio routine were two toilets. Every morning, at the same time without fail, the manager of the physio department used to go into one of the toilets with his newspaper. Every few seconds he could be heard turning a page of his newspaper. After about three to four minutes, a 'plop' sound would be heard, shortly followed by a smaller 'plop'! Soon after that would be the sound of toilet paper being sprung and torn. Then the sink tap would run for a few seconds, after which point he would come out of the toilet whistling! It was something nobody ever spoke about. Until now!

After I had done my ten minutes of standing and heard the physio manager doing his daily business, my physio would put me in my wheelchair and take me to my classroom (with my legs in callipers, sticking out straight in front of me).

In my classroom I had a wooden standing frame which had a wooden door and a belt strap preventing me from falling backwards. My physio stood me in my frame and left to me get on with my classwork. She returned an hour and a half later to get me out of the standing frame and remove my callipers. It was pure bliss every time they were taken off.

The most uncomfortable thing about standing up for so long in my callipers was that my feet used to really ache. Also, the knee pads put a lot of pressure on my knees.

I normally had a wee before having my physio and waited until my callipers came off, before going to the toilet again. On the odd occasion when I couldn't wait, my teacher took me out of my standing frame and took my callipers off, so that I could go to the toilet.

Writing about it today, it seems a bit draconian! However, it is what happened every day and it was normal for me. At that age (seven onwards), I just accepted it because it was all I knew.

In 1980, my parents bought a plot of land, a five minute drive away from where we were living, and hired an architect to design and build us a house. (I don't think architects build houses! But you know what I mean!) I remember seeing the little 3D model of our new house.

It was around this time that my parents started to argue and not get on so well.

The first time I noticed it was one Sunday when the four of us went over to Sue and Tony's house for the afternoon. When it was time to go, Dad brought Clare and I home and left Mum at

Sue and Tony's – which seemed a bit odd. Sue gave my Mum a lift home a while later.

By the time I was seven, I had outgrown my red battery-operated motorbike and received a bigger one on my seventh birthday. When I tried to use it for the first time it wasn't working properly so Dad took me to the shop to exchange it for one that was. It was white and had POLICE written in green on the front of it. And it went a bit faster than my red motorbike!

Something that I learnt to do from an early age was getting myself dressed (and undressed). It is something which has always taken me some time and energy. I've always got dressed sitting on my bed (apart from a time when I was small in Belgium, when I found it easier to get dressed sitting on the floor, leaning against my bed).

Being left handed, the left side of my body is more flexible than my right. To make the best use of my flexibility and because I cannot bend my right leg and arm as much as my left, I have always put my clothes on in the same order, dressing my right side first:

- Socks
- Pants
- Trousers
- Shoes
- T-shirt
- Jumper

Getting myself dressed is a real chore. To put my right sock on, I use my right hand to hold my leg up (with my other foot on the floor, to maintain my balance), and use my left hand to put my sock on. To get my sock on, I first hook it over my big toe and then pull the sock sideways, over the rest of my toes. I then work the rest of the sock onto my foot, by pulling each side simultaneously, until my toes are touching the end of the sock. Finally, I pull the sock over my heel.

I do the same thing in putting on my left sock; using my right hand to hold up my leg and my left hand to put on the sock.

I use the same process to put on my pants, trousers and shoes. The increased flexibility in my left leg enables me to bend and hold my leg higher than my right leg. This makes it quicker and easier to put my clothes on my left side than my right.

To pull up my trousers I stand up and balance myself, without using my crutches (which I can do for a few seconds and takes a lot of concentration). This allows me to pull my trousers up with both hands. I then fall backwards onto my bed and do my trousers up!

Getting my shoes on is the most difficult part of getting dressed and is a process in itself. First, I hold my foot up and put my shoe over the front of my foot (so that my toes are in my shoe). Then I hold and pull the back of my shoe over my heel.

My right shoe is particularly difficult to get on because I need to use both hands to pull the back of my shoe over my heel. When I don't hold it properly the back of my shoe gets crumpled underneath my heel. I then struggle to pull the back of my shoe out from underneath my heel.

It takes me twenty-five to thirty minutes to get dressed. I'm used to it because it's part of my everyday life.

I often don't pull my trousers up until I'm fully dressed and have been to the toilet. It is easier to pull and do up my trousers whilst leaning my back against the bathroom wall. The other reason is because I have to be extremely careful when I go to the toilet standing up. In doing so, I balance using only one of my crutches, which makes it very easy for me to urinate on my trousers. I have to be especially careful going to the toilet when I'm out somewhere. It can lead to embarrassing consequences – and, very occasionally, it has done!

Chapter 2

I n 1981 we moved into our new house. None of the grey-bricked inside walls had been painted yet but that didn't matter because it was fun being in our new home.

The house was bigger than our previous abode. It had a playroom along the front of the house, which led into a big square kitchen. At the other end of the kitchen were two doors. The one straight ahead went in the rectangular dining room and the other door (to the left) led into the hall.

Walking into the hall from the kitchen, you had the front door straight ahead (which was actually on the side of the house). To the left was the toilet, a study, and a little area for coats and shoes. At the end of the hall, spanning the width of the dining room, was a big lounge. The lounge had a brickbuilt, open log fireplace and big, sliding French doors, into the back garden.

In the corner of the hall were the stairs (if you were facing the living room door, the stairs were on your left). There were two flights of stairs leading up, and two flights down to the basement. The stairs doubled back on themselves – so directly below the first flight of stairs going up was the second flight of stairs to the basement. And directly below the second flight of stairs leading up was the first flight of stairs to the basement.

In the basement was a double garage, two utility rooms and a walk-in cupboard for tools.

The upstairs was split into two by a wall alongside the landing. On one side (by the stairs), was my room, Clare's room and the spare bedroom. At the other end was a separate toilet, the bathroom and my parents' bedroom.

The playroom, kitchen and dining room had French doors to the garden. Most of the downstairs floor had stone tiles. They were a creamy/light brown colour, with a hint of orange. There was carpet upstairs, on the stairs and in the living room. It was rough office carpet, leftover from my dad's office – with no underlay (you notice these things when you crawl everywhere!).

The garden was big. It was all grass. There was a bit outside the playroom, at the front of the house leading up to the road. The grass stretched along the side of the house, outside the kitchen and dining room. On the opposite side of the house was the front door and the driveway to the garage.

The back garden was huge. Outside the lounge was a square of level grass with a wooden border. Then the garden went down the hill and in the distance were a row of trees. Our garden ended somewhere before the row of trees.

Dad had a sit on lawnmower to cut the grass. He was reluctant at first but, eventually, he let me have a go on it! It had a kind of cruise control. Dad set the speed and off I went. All I had to do was steer it with its big steering wheel. I loved going on that machine. It was massive. I didn't go very fast on it but that didn't matter to me. I could go to the bottom of the garden and used to go on the mower for ages. The only issue was I didn't know how to stop it – which became a bit of a problem when I wanted to get off!

Our front door was also fun because it never had a handle on the outside. To close the door when we went out, it was a case of wrapping your hand around on the inside of the door and pulling it shut. Of course you had to get your hand out of the way before the door closed on your fingers! I enjoyed the challenge and never hurt myself.

I'm a bit concerned that I am losing my memory. I've written over 600 words on our new house in 1981 and I'm not sure what carpet we had in the playroom! Help me! I think it was the same carpet we had elsewhere in the house. But we may have had a softer carpet in the playroom. It will remain a mystery.

Soon after we moved, Dad bought Mum a second-hand gold coloured Toyota Corona.

One of the first things I did in our new house was to teach myself a shocking lesson. As I went to bed one night my bedside lamp wasn't working. Liking to know how things work and to fix them, I started to investigate. The light build felt wobbly so I thought there must be problem with the light fitting. I unscrewed the light build and gave it a little shake, which sounded alright. I then wanted to see if the light fitting was wobbly so I stuck my index finger in it! It was my first experience of an electric shock and it made me burst out crying. Mum hurried up the stairs, asking, "What have you done?"

I learned not do that again! In my defence, I was seven years old. (My lamp just needed a new light bulb.)

Our dog, Zebedee, was fully grown and clearly now was the animal leader of the house. Peter obviously had had enough of Zebedee bullying him and sniffing his butt because the cat took it upon himself to find somewhere else to live.

Clare went looking for Peter, after he had disappeared, for two or three days. It didn't take Clare long to find him. Peter had moved in with an old couple who lived three houses away from us. It was a hot and sunny day and their garage door was open (at the front of the house), where Clare spotted Peter asleep in a cat basket. The old couple really enjoyed looking after Peter so we let them keep him.

In our new house, the stairs were different to the ones in our old house. The steps on the new staircase had backs to them. No longer could I crawl up the stairs by holding the back of each step and pulling myself up the stairs. I had to adapt and find another way to crawl up them.

I quickly learnt to do so by using the strength in my arms. I put both of my hands flat on the third step above the one I was kneeling on, held my arms out straight and pushed down on my hands. It took a bit more effort than in our old house. However, it didn't stop me from crawling up the stairs pretty quickly.

Also, because the stairs were carpeted (with a bit of rough carpet), it caused more friction on my knees and legs. I couldn't glide down the stairs as freely as I did in our old house.

The wooden staircase banister was created by two horizontal strips of pine coloured wood, measuring about ten inches wide. One strip of wood ran along (and formed) the top of the banister, while the second strip ran along halfway between the floor and the top strip of wood. The banister was held together by a series of wooden upright posts, at roughly fifty centimetre intervals. I like mixing together my units of measurements!

The same banister design continued upstairs, all around the landing. The length of the landing ran parallel to the length of the downstairs hallway. The two gaps between the strips of wood along the banister were big enough to fit my head through – but not my whole body!

I'll come back upstairs shortly. I'm needed elsewhere at the moment.

Something that I became interested in, and liked playing with, was our open log fire in the living room. I found it slightly mesmerising and enjoyed moving the burning logs about with the big black fire tongs and poker we had. I liked the thrill of boy versus fire – I think my caveman instincts came into play!

One day when I was sitting watching TV in the lounge, I kept looking at the burning logs on the fire. I became more interested by the fire than the programme I was watching and decided the fire needed another log on it – and the logs that were already on the fire needed to be moved a bit first.

I crawled over and knelt in front of the fireplace. One of the burning logs was on top of the other one. Using the long poker I pushed the bottom log towards the back of the fireplace but, for some reason, this made the top log roll off of the fire and fall onto the carpet!

In my defence, I was only seven or eight and didn't know the laws of physics yet. *Oh no! Oh no!* I thought. *What do I do? What do I do?*

I looked around and saw the basket of magazines to my right. For a moment I thought I could pick up the smouldering log and put it back on the fire and nobody would know about it!

I grabbed one of the magazines and wrapped one of its inside pages around the log and picked it up with my hand. But it was far too hot and I dropped it back onto the carpet!

It was at this point that Mum walked into the lounge and shouted "WHAT THE HELL ARE YOU DOING?" As she came over she said, "MOVE AWAY FROM THE FIRE."

With the tongs she put the log back on the fire.

Feeling taken aback I said sheepishly "I was only trying to put another log on the fire..."

Mum: "LOOK AT WHAT YOU'VE DONE TO THE CARPET. YOU KNOW NOT TO PLAY WITH THE FIRE."

There were now several big black burn marks on the carpet. At least it was office carpet, which probably wasn't as flammable as domestic carpet!

Me: "I'm sorry."

Mum picked me up and smacked me on the bum and carried me upstairs to my bedroom.

Mum: "I can't believe what you've done."

Me: "I'm sorry."

(Pause)

Me: "I've burnt my hand. It really hurts."

Mum dumped me on my bed.

Mum: "Show me your hand."

Mum (looking at my hand): "Well, you can sit here and think about your hand and about what you've done."

Mum slammed my bedroom door on her way out.

I felt sorry because my hand was really painful. (I didn't know at the time that toothpaste is a really good thing to put on burns.)

I was pleased that it was Mum who caught me, and not Dad. However, I think Dad had already moved out at that point. Had he been there I don't think I would have played with the fire because he would have hit the roof.

Mum sometimes referred to me as being 'a little sod' when I was young because I often did things I wasn't meant to do! My day as a pyromaniac was over. (I told you that I would be back upstairs soon!)

By 1981, it wasn't uncommon for my parents to argue with each other. Within a few months after moving into our new house, Dad moved out and into an apartment, with his new girlfriend, Yvonne, and her daughter, Juliet.

At home, nothing much really changed because, for the past few years, Dad hadn't been around much in the evenings anyway. Mum sometimes became resentful of Dad (and Yvonne). From time to time, Mum would say something like, "It's alright for your Dad, he can afford it." I began to feel sorry for Mum.

Another thing Mum didn't like, were our cheap kitchen cupboards because they had thin doors, which were difficult to slide open and closed.

Once Dad moved out, Clare and I spent every Sunday with him, Yvonne and Juliet. On Sundays Clare and I would get up and we always watched *d'Artagnan and The Three Musketeers* on TV, before Dad came to pick us up at 9.30 am.

I enjoyed spending Sundays with Dad. Unlike before, Sundays became different from other days of the week. We would spend all day with him. If the weather was okay, we would go out somewhere. If it rained we would normally stay in and play cards and other games. Dad taught me backgammon, which I still like playing today.

I remember meeting Juliet when I was eight and she was five. Clare and I got on well with her. Clare always got on better with Yvonne than I did (and I think they're still in touch with each other today). Yvonne and I got on alright together but I found her a bit too strict and domineering. I got the sense that she slightly resented the time that Dad spent with me and she would rather have had him all to herself. Every now and again, Yvonne was a bit rude and secretive. We would be sat around the table eating diner when Yvonne would suddenly start a conversation with Dad in German! Yvonne was a cigarette chain smoker and she liked her beer and whisky!

Dad brought Clare and I home after dinner on Sundays, he would light up a big fat cigar on the way. Before leaving his apartment, he would often find some dark, creamy Belgian chocolate lurking around somewhere.

When we got home, Dad would sometimes go into the lounge, shut the door and start arguing with Mum. This was a bit upsetting. I always felt protective of Mum because she gave the impression that Dad was 'the big bad wolf'.

Dad often brought us back with some leftover food in tinfoil for Zebedee that they (him, Yvonne and Juliet) hadn't eaten during the week. On one occasion, Mum unwrapped three uncooked steaks – so we had steak for dinner the next day!

Here's an example of the slightly different approach my parents each had of encouraging me to do things for myself.

At meal times on Sundays I was always given a curved (bowl-like) plate (so that I didn't get food on the tablecloth), whilst everyone else had a normal plate. If I had difficulty cutting my meat, Dad would do it for me. Whereas at home, Mum's attitude was, "You can cut your own food up and don't get any of it on the table!" (We weren't posh enough to have a tablecloth at home!)

One of my Dad's favourite sayings has always been, "Un Souiljaert n'a jamais mal" (a Souiljaert never feels pain).

One Sunday afternoon, while play-fighting with Dad on their lounge floor, the little finger on my left hand got bent right back. Throughout the rest of the afternoon and evening, as it turned a blue-green colour, I was moaning that my finger was really hurting. Dad was like, "Un Souiljaert n'a jamais mal. Arrête d'être un bébé" (stop being a baby).

The next morning my finger was still hurting so Mum took me to the hospital – only to discover that it was broken. No, not the hospital, my finger! The hospital put a blue and grey splint on my finger and wrapped a bandage around my hand to keep it in place.

Imagine the delight I had telling Dad that my finger was broken and that he was the one who broke it! I remember his comeback was something like, "Well, there's nothing much you can do to help mend a broken finger!"

A month or two after my parents split up, Sue and Tony also separated – and Sue, Jane and Ian moved back to Devon in England. I was a bit disappointed to see Jane leave.

This was followed shortly by Mary leaving her husband and moving into the newly built house next door to us. Mary, from America, lived in Embourg and was in the circle of English-speaking friends with Mum and Sue.

Mary had two sons, Jack and Douglas, aged eleven and three respectively. Clare and I used to go and play with them. They had one of those early tennis, bat and ball game consoles that plugged into the TV, which was good fun.

Do you remember the first record you bought? I bought mine in 1981; 'Every Little Thing She Does Is Magic' by The Police, which is a great uplifting song.

People say you like the music that your parents listened to when you were growing up. This is certainly true for me.

In our lounge was the same stereo that was in our old house, which Dad wasn't keen on me touching. Mum was happy for me to use it now. I liked listening to the radio and remember hearing Steve Wright on Radio Luxembourg. I used to wonder how, playing vinyl records, radio DJs knew when to stop talking over the start of songs.

I didn't use the record player in the lounge myself, because I hadn't yet mastered how to put the needle on the record. Being left handed, I found it difficult to do at first because my hand obscured where the needle should go at the start of the record.

However, I liked the records Mum played:

- Saturday Night Fever
- The Beatles – 'Please Please Me'
- Paul Simon – 'One-Trick Pony' (which includes my very favourite Paul Simon song 'Late in the evening')
- Paul Simon – 'Still Crazy After All These Years'
- Neil Diamond – 'The Jazz Singer'

Clare liked the *Grease* soundtrack (no surprise there!).

In the car Dad often played a tape by French singer Francis Cabrel, I've got that album too, now, and like every song on it.

(Wait a second – this isn't a book about music. Just think of it as a music break. I'm going back upstairs now.)

Because I didn't know how to walk yet, whenever I went to the toilet, I always sat down on it to do a wee. It was while I was sitting on the loo upstairs one day that I had an epiphany. (Many ideas have come to me when I've been to the toilet over the years. It's due to the mind being relaxed.)

I was used to standing up and holding onto things. However, I suddenly realised that I could stand up – and using the toilet wall and doorframe – I could reach out and grab hold of the banister on the landing.

So I stood up and put my left hand on the toilet wall to balance myself. I then started to step to the right, outside the toilet. When I got outside the toilet, I moved my left hand and held onto the doorframe. All I had to do then was to keep stepping to the right until I could reach and grab hold of the banister with my right hand. *I knew I could do it.* I just hadn't done it before.

The key thing was not to let go of the doorframe with my left hand. I kept slowly stepping to my right until both of my arms were stretched out and I touched the banister with my right hand. Once I did so, I was home and dry.

It was then just a case of closing my right hand and holding onto the banister. I could then let go of the doorframe, and take bigger steps to the right, until I could hold onto the banister with both hands.

Walking sideways along the banister was a doddle because I had done it before. At the end of the landing was a ninety degree turn to the right, which I had also walked around before. When I reached the stairs I got on my knees and crawled down the stairs.

Every morning from then on when I got up and dressed, I crawled to the landing and, holding onto the banister with both hands, I pulled myself up and walked to the toilet. I would then walk to the top of the stairs and crawl down them.

In the evenings, I would crawl up the stairs, pull myself up using the banister and walk to the toilet. The bathroom was next door to the toilet. I could walk from the toilet into the bathroom using the doorframes as support. I walked around the bathroom by leaning on the walls.

It was a matter of weeks after my epiphany sitting on the toilet that I had another great idea. It was Saturday morning, I had got dressed and been to the toilet, Mum and Clare were downstairs somewhere. After walking around the landing to the top of the stairs, I thought, *why don't I walk down the stairs?*

Walking around the banister upstairs was something I now did without thinking. The banister on the stairs was the same banister that was around the landing, it was just at an angle.

I was a bit scared I might fall down the stairs but I knew that if I didn't let go of the banister, I wouldn't fall. I thought about calling out to Mum to come and stand by me, just in case, but I wanted to see if I could walk down the stairs by myself first – and I absolutely knew that I could do it.

So I went for it. Very slowly and carefully I walked down the stairs sideways. I put my right foot down on the first step. It immediately became obvious that I needed to put my right foot as far over to the right as possible, and on the edge of the step, for there to be enough room on the step for my left foot. It wasn't an issue. With each step I took, I thought *this is so easy*. And my confidence grew.

When I got down the first flight of stairs I was amazed at how easily and quickly I did it. I thought, *is that all there is to it? Why haven't I done it sooner?*

Felling pretty elated, in excitement, I called out "Mum, Mum come and look at this…"

She appeared and said, "What have you done?" "Look at what I can do…" I replied.

I turned 180 degrees and very carefully walked down the second flight of stairs. Mum was amazed and gave me a kiss well done.

The funny thing is, all I wanted to do when I reached the bottom of the stairs was to carry on walking but I had nothing to walk with!

I was eight or nine years old at the time. Writing about it now, I find it baffling why the physios I had at school in Belgium never gave me anything to walk with. All they made me do was to stand in my heavy and uncomfortable callipers every day.

It didn't take me long to learn to walk up the stairs. It was the same as walking down them – only in reverse!

Walking up and down the stairs became normal to me. It wasn't quicker than crawling but I preferred to walk. This was partly due to the rough carpet and the friction it caused on my hands, knees and legs when I crawled.

I have never fallen when walking up or down stairs. This is because I have always done so in a very controlled manner.

I still crawled around downstairs. However, I started to walk around holding onto things. It was like a game to me. Mapping out in my mind how I could get from A to B. There were lots of things I used to lean on, balance against and grab hold of; walls, doorframes, doors, radiators, tables, chairs and any sturdy objects. I could walk from and to anywhere in the house.

For example, to go from the playroom to the lounge I went across the kitchen, through the dining room, into the lounge. (However, I don't think of this as 'proper walking'. I didn't start to walk properly until we moved back to England in April 1984.)

Every morning before school, Clare and I sat at the kitchen table and had some cereal. Mum would then get the cutlery tray, out of the kitchen drawer, and the cutlery holder from the dishwasher, for me to put the clean eating-irons in the tray – whilst Clare unstacked the rest of the dishwasher. I always used to say it would be a lot easier, when they (Mum and Clare) stacked the dishwasher if they put each type of cutlery in separate compartments of the holder but Mum and Clare disagreed with me!

I still had the same slightly unfriendly taxi driver (Francois) taking me to and from school. By 1982 he had a new white Mercedes. (White had become the standard colour of taxis in Liege. I think it's a bit racist, if you ask me!) Francois often had the radio on which I enjoyed listening to.

In the taxi I always sat in back on the left. Sitting next to me was a girl called Dominique. She had light brown hair and walked like Forrest Gump (with callipers).

It was in 1982 when Dominique and I started holding hands on the way to and from school. We had a little kiss sometimes as well! The song 'Only You' by Yazoo reminds me of her because it was in the charts at the time. However, at school, Dominique was more interested in another boy. She was obviously a little player!

At school, my physio got me riding a blue tricycle that had a foot holder on each pedal. When I first started riding it, I went a bit too fast around corners and one of the stabilisers would often be up in the air. People told me to slow down but I didn't! I rode it round the school playground. I could ride my tricycle much faster than my motorbike!

My reading and writing (in French) was improving slightly. Every morning in class, for what felt like an eternity and quickly became boring, we had to copy from the blackboard, days of the week, for example:

Hier c'était Mardi Aujourd'hui c'est Mercredi Demain sera Jeudi

Logically, and to encompass every shool-day, you only need to write the above for five days. However, my class must have been writing the same thing, on a five day cycle, for months.

This led on to something a little more advanced – writing different verbs and word endings for each of the below (I must have written hundreds of different verbs).

Je
Tu
Il
Elle
Nous
Vous
Ils
Elles

Because my handwriting was big and wobbly, like a few people in my class, I used an electric typewriter. My handwriting has improved over the years but it's still wobbly!

Up until I was eight or nine, I didn't know how to pronounce hard C and G sounds; I used to say *toffee* instead of *coffee* and *darden* instead of *garden*. My speech therapist at school taught me to use the back of my throat to articulate C and G sounds. At first I found it difficult and unnatural but I soon got used to it.

Now, I find it virtually impossible to say 'darden'!

Mum hoped that having speech therapy would stop me dribbling. But it didn't. Although by 1982 I wasn't dribbling 100% of the time. Especially not on the way to and from school, holding hands with, and kissing Dominique!

In 1983 I fractured my skull at school.

Inside my school was a long slope down to the dining room. The dining room had double doors which led out to the playground and to some prefab classrooms (where mine was). Directly outside the dining room was a terrace area, followed by tarmac, which went downhill to the playground and my classroom.

To eliminate a step between the terrace area and the start of the tarmac was a strip of concrete. In the middle of the concrete were two shoeprints (obviously someone had stepped onto the concrete, before it had dried, when it had been laid years earlier).

If the dining room doors were open, I could maintain a decent speed down the long slope in my wheelchair, out of the dining room and down the hill to my classroom.

It was a warm and sunny afternoon when the Prince and Princess of Belgium (don't ask me which prince and princess, I have no idea) were making an appearance at the conference centre next door to my school. My class was one of the ones who were let out to briefly go and see the monarchs.

On returning to school that afternoon I was feeling really good. It was a nice day and I had just met the Prince and Princess. So I decided to try and break my record of how fast I could go down the long slope, through the dining room and down the hill back to my classroom.

My challenge started off really well. I whizzed down the long slope and out of the dining room at breakneck speed. What I didn't envisage was one of the little front wheels of my wheelchair getting caught in one of the concrete footprints, my wheelchair overturning and me getting knocked unconscious.

Instead of breaking my record I broke my head!

I remember coming in and out of consciousness while lying on one of the dining room tables, with people standing round me. I came in and out of consciousness again in an ambulance. When I woke up, I found myself in a hospital bed.

As I opened my eyes, I saw Mum, Dad and Clare sitting next to my bed. The first thing I thought was: *Why are Mum and Dad sitting next to each other and not arguing?*

Shortly after I fully regained consciousness I started vomiting severely. One of the nurses recommended that Coke was good at reducing sickness so Mum went and bought me a few cans and I felt better.

I only stayed in hospital for a few days, before coming home and going to back to school. For about the next month I wore a brown leather helmet to protect my head from getting any more bumps. When I returned to school, the two concrete shoeprints had been filled in.

I've got a very strong head and am used to falling on it!

When Clare and I went to the supermarket with Mum I used to enjoy looking at all of the seven inch records which were in the charts and sometimes I bought one! I remember buying 'I won't let you down' by PhD.

On my ninth birthday I got a little record player which I used in my bedroom. I could now practice putting the needle on seven inch records. I overcame the issue of my left hand being an obstruction. It didn't take me long to learn to align the needle with the start of the record. I then pressed the 'on' button, which started the record spinning, and used the little lever which lowered the needle onto the record. It was easy.

Once I received my record player I regularly bought a record and also played the old ones Mum had. However, I couldn't stand the one she had by Kate Bush – 'Wuthering Heights'. Every time I heard it on the radio I put my hands over my ears!

Today, I recognise that Kate Bush is a good song writer but I still don't like her high-pitched squeaky tones and she wears too much make-up!

The first album I got was Michael Jackson's 'Thriller'. Surely one of the best pop albums ever? I know it's subjective and probably a generational thing!

The toys I had in the playroom over the years were Lego, Playmobil and a train set. I obviously liked building things and they were all good toys for enhancing my dexterity. When I first got the train set I found putting two pieces of train track together very fiddly. However, like everything in life, I persisted and it soon became a piece of cake! Our long playroom was good for building a big train track. I liked my train set because it was electric and mechanical – and something that I built myself.

Occasionally, as a treat, we would spend the night in the playroom. Clare and I had a TV in there and we used to like watching *CHiPs* and *The Incredible Hulk*. I must have been eight or nine when I went to a fancy dress birthday party as the Incredible Hulk (I developed big biceps and arms at a young age from crawling around everywhere).

Mum did a really good job at dressing me up; she made strategic rips in an old pair of trousers and in an old shirt and painted my body green! I remember riding my blue tricycle outside during the party and people saying I looked really good.

When we got home after the party I went upstairs to have a bath. I was really surprised and disappointed when I looked in the mirror. All of the green paint had come off of my chin due to me dribbling. However even that, nor Mum always nagging me, stopped me dribbling.

There was no school on Wednesday afternoons in Belgium. When I arrived home at lunchtime, we would have something to eat and then Clare and I would go to a local art and crafts club.

Taking into consideration my wobbly handwriting, I've never been one for drawing or painting so I opted to do pottery. I made lots of things out of clay but my speciality was making mugs and cups. However, most of the ones I made seemed to have a leverage problem. I wasn't the best at thinning out the clay properly, which made my mugs rather thick and heavy. Hence, the handles had a tendency to fall off of my mugs, the first time someone drank out of them! I improved over time but I'm no Patrick Swayze.

I'm Patrick Souiljaert.

My tenth birthday was on a Monday. Unbeknown to me, the day before, while Clare and I were at Dad's, Mum painted my bedroom in a sea blue colour. When I went to bed that night she sneakily ensured that I didn't turn on my bedroom light. It was a nice surprise when I woke up on my birthday.

During the school holidays, three times a year, Mum, Clare and I normally went back to England and stayed either with Nan and Grandad or with my aunt and uncle, and my three cousins, in

Shoreham-by-Sea. We were a close family and Mum got on extremely well with her sister Liz, and John, my uncle.

Clare and I got on well with our cousins, who are older than me; Damian by eight years, Keith by six years and Becky by eighteen months. Clare and Becky got on particularly well with each other.

We always went in the car to England by going on the Townsend Thoresen ferry, from Zeebrugge to Dover. We got to know the ferry crossing very well. It often took more than four and a half hours on a choppy day and I wasn't very good when it came to seasickness! At least there was a film to watch during the journey. On virtually every crossing we went on, they showed *The Cannonball Run*. Clare and I loved that film and got to know every line in it!

In the 1970s Liz and John (and my cousins) lived in a houseboat on Shoreham Beach (not literally on the beach! Shoreham Beach is an area in Shoreham-by-Sea). It was the same houseboat that Leo Sayer once lived in.

I remember, at that time, Liz and John had a white Peugeot estate, with an eight track cassette player. Liz had Simon & Garfunkel's 1969 live album and used to play it in the car. In 1980 Liz and John bought, and moved into, a five bed detached house nearby.

When we went to stay with Liz and John – and we went out somewhere – I always asked Damian to push me (in my buggy) because he did so like a madman! I would say to him, "Faster, faster... Go faster!" Damian would tip the buggy up, and go round corners, on one wheel. It always made me laugh a lot. On one occasion, one of the wheels snapped off of the buggy!

When we got a bit older Damian and I had wrestling matches. I've always had strong arms, but with him being eight years older than me, Damian was always stronger than I was. Damian would get both of my hands behind my back and say "Surrender..."

Although it was quite painful I always replied, "Never..." but eventually I had to do so, reluctantly!

Don't worry; I got my own back on Damian when he started body-slamming me! I quickly became wise to this and I rolled out of the way at the last second. Damian would then slam down onto the floor and hurt himself. This gave me the opportunity to body-slam Damian!

Once I had learnt to walk up and down the stairs at home in Belgium, I learnt to do the same when we stayed in England. The stairs in Nan and Grandad's maisonette were pretty easy. They had a rail on the wall however it didn't go right to the bottom of the stairs. When I walked down the stairs and reached the end of the rail, I just leaned on the wall or used the banister on the other side to walk down the last few steps.

Liz and John's house had three bedrooms downstairs, used by my cousins – so I slept in the spare room upstairs. The stairs there were a little more tricky because they had a sharp turn in them (making three of the steps very narrow). However, I found a way to walk up and down the stairs.

I have never come across a set of stairs I couldn't negotiate because there's always something for me to hold onto, or a wall to lean against to support myself. Whenever I come across some new stairs I think, *how am I going to get up them?* I can always find a way of achieving something when I put my mind to it.

John, my uncle, was a journalist and in the early eighties he got a job in Hong Kong. This led Liz, John and my cousins to move to Hong Kong and to rent out their house on Shoreham Beach.

In 1984 it was arranged that Mum, Clare and I would move back to England and live in Liz and John's house. We already knew people in Shoreham and it was a nice place to live.

The date was set, we were moving on 1st April 1984.

As I had never been taught to read and write in English before, a few months prior to moving to England, Mum started to teach me how to read in English. It was difficult, for Mum at least, because I wasn't very interested in learning to read.

I remember sitting on the living room floor and Mum having all these rectangular flashcards. Each card contained one word. Mum went through each word and put the cards on the floor, and said to me, "Now make a sentence using some of the cards." But all I wanted to do was play music on the stereo!

However, Mum did get me to read *Jonathan Livingston Seagull*. It was the first book I ever read. I've never been good at reading books and I've only ever read a handful of them (literally). I have started to read lots of books but quickly get bored with them.

I find it funny how I developed a wide vocabulary from reading so few books. I will reveal how I have done so later in this book.

When we went out somewhere, it wasn't uncommon for Mum to leave me in the car for a few minutes while she popped into a shop. One time, shortly before we moved back to England, something happened that really scared me. It seemed like Mum had been gone for absolutely ages and I didn't know which shop she had gone to. I started to worry that something had happened to her and she wasn't going to come back. I wanted to go and look for her but the keys were in the ignition and I could hardly go crawling on the road. I felt like I was trapped. It was very strange because I hadn't experienced that fear before. It was such a relief when she returned to the car. The fear I had been feeling for about five minutes quickly disappeared.

Leading up to April, for some reason my school gave me a new tricycle. It was dark green and was absolutely massive. Oddly, something on the pedal mechanism was back to front. To go forwards I had to pedal backwards! It didn't matter because I got used to it.

The bike was so big that Dad came to pick it, and me, up in the Range Rover. It was the first time that Dad had ever picked me up from school. It was a real treat.

A few days before we moved, Mum said that she was going to buy me a computer in England because she said it would be good for me. This excited me. The only exposure I had had to a computer, up to this point, was to the early Apple computer in my classroom.

My abiding memory of school in Belgium is standing in my standing frame with my callipers on, using my electric typewriter. My only regret is I didn't learn to read and write in French properly. Other than that, je ne regrette rien.

I was a little sad we were moving because we wouldn't spend Sundays with Dad anymore but I was really excited about moving to England. Although I spoke fluent French, at home with Mum and Clare we always spoke English and it was our first language. I was looking forward to living in a country where everybody spoke English.

Clare was more upset to be leaving Belgium than I was. She has always been a bit closer to Dad than I have. Also, with Clare being two years older than me, at school in Belgium she had been taught how to read and write in French properly.

Clare has always had more of an affinity with France and speaking French, and Dad had moved there in the late eighties. In 2007 Clare moved to France and now lives near Dad.

I've always had a difference of opinion with Clare when it comes to our nationality. Before my parents lived in Bromley, they spent a spell in Antwerp, where Clare was born. Therefore, Clare considers herself Belgian and has a Belgian passport, whereas I'm English/British and have a UK passport!

On 30th March 1984 – two days before we were due to move – Mum received a phone call from Mandy (one of our new neighbours who lived a few doors away from Liz and John's house). Mandy had been to see the people who were due to move out of Liz and John's house, to get the keys from them, only to be told that they had no intention of moving out! They became known as 'the squatters'.

What could we do?

Everything else was organised; the removal guys had already arrived and were busy packing up all of our things, Clare and I were due to start at our new schools after the Easter holidays.

There was nothing we could do about it so we moved as planned on 1st April 1984.

Two other things happened on that day in history:

- Dad, Yvonne and Juliet moved into Zebedee's house!
- Marvin Gaye was shot dead by his father, following a dispute.

It was while on the ferry, somewhere between Zeebrugge and Dover, that I made a decision. I'm going to a new school, I thought. I don't know anyone there, it would help me if I stop dribbling – and I should start practising to do so right now.

And it was then and there that I stopped dribbling.

Chapter 3

Mum, Clare and I arrived in Shoreham on the evening of 1st April and we stayed with Mandy and George for the first four days.

Mandy and George were an elderly couple and part of a family of friends we knew in Shoreham. They had quite a big house and it was on the opposite side of the road, and a few houses down, from Liz and John's house – which was currently occupied by the squatters.

Mandy and George's garden backed onto the beach and every year, on 5th November, they hosted a bonfire party.

After staying with Mandy and George, we rented a two bedroom, second floor flat on the seafront. Clare and I had to share a room but it wasn't a big deal. I hadn't expected that I was going to need to tackle stairs when we moved back to England because I was going to have one of the downstairs bedrooms in Liz and John's house.

However, I was used to climbing stairs and it was no big deal – and we weren't going to be living there for very long. I say it was no big deal but it did take a bit of energy and effort. With it being a second floor flat, there were four flights of stairs.

I climbed them like the stairs in our house in Belgium – walking sideways, holding onto the banister rail. The stairs were wooden and weren't carpeted but each step had a little lip on it. On the plus side, it made climbing the stairs a bit easier than I was used to because there was no carpet friction. On the negative side, I had to learn to move each foot out a bit, to avoid getting my feet caught under the lip of every step.

Once I got used to the stairs up to our flat, I timed myself to see how fast I could get up or down them each time! I didn't climb the stairs all of the time; sometimes Mum or Clare carried me.

I always think of 1984 as the year we moved back to England and am fond of the music that was in the charts in that year. There are three songs in particular which resonate with me: Duran Duran – 'The Reflex.' Thompson Twins – 'Hold Me Now' Nik Kershaw – 'Wouldn't It Be Good'

Whenever I hear one of these songs now, I always think of the time we moved back to England and were living in the second floor flat because the songs were being played a lot on the radio at that time.

I also remember the weather in April, May and June of 1984 being nice and sunny. I wonder if Michael Fish is still around to confirm this for me? No, on second thoughts, Michael Fish said there wasn't going to be a hurricane in 1987. I'm better off asking Ian McCaskill!

Once we moved back to England, Clare and I spoke to Dad roughly every seven to ten days. Mum would always get us to reverse the call charges because she said we couldn't afford to phone abroad – and he could afford it. (With my good memory for numbers, I will never forget the full international number (13 digits) we used to call Dad in 1984.)

I found it a bit frustrating speaking with Dad on the phone because it would often be, what I class as a, 'hello, how are you conversation' It would go something like this (in French):

Dad: "How are you?"

Me: "I'm alright. How are you?"

Dad: "I'm okay. How's school?"

Me: "It's alright. How's work?"

Dad: "Not bad…"

Our conversations didn't seem to have much substance. But it was my fault as much as Dad's.

Educationally, I started at my new middle school, which was only a five minute drive from our flat. As Clare had turned twelve years old a week before we moved back to England, she attended Buckingham Park School, in Shoreham, for the summer term of 1984, and went to school by bus. Unlike in Belgium, my school day was shorter than Clare's – which was good!

The first thing that I found a little strange was that I had to wear a school uniform (and a tie). As a ten-year-old boy I thought a tie was only something you wore to work. My uniform consisted of grey trousers, a grey jumper with a yellow stripe around the V-neck collar and a yellow stripe around the bottom of the jumper, a white or grey shirt and a grey tie with thin diagonal yellow stripes on it. It didn't take me long to learn how to do up my tie.

My school was an ordinary school with, what was known at the time as, a PH (physically handicapped) unit, called Pebbles.

I went to school by taxi and my taxi driver was a massive bloke called Tiny! He drove a maroon Volvo hatchback. Tiny always had the local radio station Southern Sound on in the car, which I liked listening to.

At school I had a grey DHSS manual wheelchair to get around in.

The first few days at school were a bit scary. I was shy and a bit quiet because I didn't know anyone or what to expect. Because I couldn't read or write very well I was put in a class with kids a year younger than me. I didn't mind it that much but it did feel a bit strange. Some of my lessons were with my class in the main school but most of the time I was in a small group of people, who were being taught in Pebbles.

I soon made friends with Richard and Justin Smith (brothers) and Matthew Atwater – not forgetting Martin, who defied the odds. They all had Duchenne Muscular Dystrophy (MD) and used electric wheelchairs.

Duchenne MD is a genetic condition, due to a defective gene, that causes muscles to progressively waste and weaken. The Duchenne strain of MD only affects boys and they are lucky to live past their teenage years. It makes me feel grateful that I have CP – which is not life-threatening.

Richard and Justin were always happy and smiling. Richard was a year older, whilst Justin a year younger, than me. Matthew was wise for his age at ten, and tended to moan about things like the state of the school and of the country (although I think I'm remembering Matthew when he was twelve or thirteen). Martin was also the same age as me and I got on particularly well with him. Martin didn't care much for rules and we often had a laugh.

I also had friends from my class in the main school. I was friends with Paul , James, Joanne and Anya. Anya was very bright for a nine-year-old.

Most of my lessons in Pebbles were with a girl my age called Zoe, who didn't appear to be disabled and who was often a bit unruly and naughty. Zoe didn't seem to have much respect for Mrs Nightingale who was in charge of Pebbles. Mrs Nightingale was an old lady about to retire that summer. She had curly grey hair and wore glasses – and she sometimes farted!

One incident I remember was when a small group of us were sitting waiting for Mrs Nightingale to come and start the lesson. Zoe decided to stand up, went over to the whiteboard and drew a cartoon-like picture of Mrs Nightingale, with her curly hair and glasses – and with wind coming out of her bottom!

As we heard Mrs Nightingale coming, Zoe picked up the board rubber and started trying to rub her picture off the board. However, she had used a red indelible pen and her picture wasn't disappearing! As Mrs Nightingale's footsteps got louder and louder Zoe became more and more frantic, trying to erase her drawing – but she couldn't get rid of it. I felt sorry for Mrs Nightingale because she often found it hard keeping Zoe under control.

One of the first things that happened when I started at my new school, was to get rid of my callipers. When I took in my heavy and uncomfortable callipers from Belgium, my new physio, Anne, took one look at them and said, "They look like something from the dark ages to me. I would throw them away if I were you."

Can you imagine how I felt?

I had worn and stood in my callipers, for hours every day at school, for the last three years and my new physio dismissed them straightaway. I felt great. I was never going to wear those horrible things again. (Anne did say my hips were very strong and I will never know if that was due to wearing my callipers for so long.)

Anne started my walking career! She gave me a rollator (a zimmer frame with two wheels at the front of it), and off I went.

The first mistake I made with my rollator was to try and walk too fast with it. Imagine what happens to someone walking on a treadmill when the treadmill is set too fast. That was me with my new rollator! I could push it faster than I could walk with it! It was a good way to learn that I needed to walk slowly with it. At first I only walked some of the time. I needed to teach myself how to walk and build up my stamina.

Pebbles had its own little playground and I went slowly walking around it at break times. The playground was mainly concreted and it had a couple of slopes. There was also an area of grass, which had a tent on it, but I tended to keep off the grass because it was difficult to push the rollator on it.

Walking up the slopes wasn't too bad. However, walking down the slopes was difficult and scary at first. I had to hold the rollator back and walk very slowly down the slopes. The rollator was quite heavy and stopping it from going too fast down the slopes was hard to do. The playground had a little step and it was a bit tricky to get the rollator up it to start with but I worked out a way to do it; by lifting the left wheel of the rollator up the step first, followed by the right wheel.

It wasn't long before my strength, stamina and confidence grew and I was walking more and more. Walking gave me a new lease of life and a sense of freedom and I much preferred it to crawling everywhere. However, my rollator wasn't much use to me walking up and down the stairs at our seafront flat! Mum and Clare used to leave the rollator at the top and bottom of the stairs for me.

Sometimes when walking with the rollator (and walking in general), it wasn't uncommon for me to start to feel myself falling backwards or sideways. To correct my balance I would just grab hold of the rollator and pull on it slightly. It became an unconscious reflex.

Anne was also the first person that I defied in life. Shortly after she started me walking, she predicted that I wouldn't be able to walk past the age of eighteen. She believed the bones in my legs wouldn't be strong enough to support me.

All I can say now, at forty years old, is that I think I will still be walking when I'm eighty.

An issue which became apparent when I started at school in England was that I had nothing to write with! At school in Belgium I had all my lessons in the same classroom and I used an electric typewriter. Because I now had some lessons in my main school class and others in Pebbles, I needed something I could carry around with me.

The solution was to buy a portable Brother typewriter (which Dad paid for). I got on really well with my new Brother! I thought it was really high tech; it was electronic and had a little LCD display. Although it was portable I did find it a bit heavy and I had to be careful not to bang or drop it. I put it in my rucksack, which I carried around on the handles on the back of my wheelchair. It was difficult for me to get my bag on and off my wheelchair so people would help me do so.

One thing I found hard throughout my school years was pushing myself in my wheelchair. Although I've always had strong arms, my coordination is a bit poor. To easily push yourself in a wheelchair you need good coordination. This is the reason why you never see people with severe CP playing wheelchair basketball or doing a marathon.

In hindsight having an electric wheelchair or scooter at school would have made my life a lot easier. I've never been a fan of wheelchairs and I'll explain why later in this book.

One thing I was good at in my class was mental arithmetic. The teacher, Mrs Orange, often gave us a ten question, quick fire, mental arithmetic test. She first got everyone to write the question numbers in their exercise book and then she said things like '7x8', '63÷9', '78+11', '56–13'.

Because I was using my electronic typewriter, I couldn't write the question numbers beforehand. Hence, after typing the answer to each question, I also had to hit the 'return' key, followed by typing the next question number, a dot and then a space. This gave me less thinking time than everybody else, to work out the answer to each question. However, it didn't matter because it still gave me enough time to work out each calculation.

In the main school corridor were some BBC B computers. I did go on one sometimes. However, they weren't well maintained and therefore tended not to be used.

I had English classes with Mrs Nightingale in Pebbles. She often spoke about the magic 'e' at the end of words. She would say something like, "The magic 'e' at the end of the word changes the sound of the word…" (For example 'rate'.)

There was also 'story time' every afternoon in Pebbles. We would all sit round in a semicircle and Mrs Nightingale would read us a story. It was so babyish!

I would often go home with a Ladybird book to read – and an A4 sheet of paper asking: What was the story about? What did you like about the story? What didn't you like about the story?

I was never too enamoured reading the books (but I did read them) and Mum helped me to fill in the question sheet.

At break times in Pebbles everyone was given a half pint bottle of milk to drink. After a while, I decided I didn't want to have half a pint of warm milk, which had been sitting in the sun for ages, anymore. For some reason I didn't want Mum to know about it. So I came up with a cunning plan!

At home, on the side of the kitchen table was Mum's manual typewriter and a small tray of utility letters etc. One evening after dinner, I typed a note for Pebbles and put Mum's name on the bottom of it. The only issue was I didn't know how to spell 'sincerely' – but I knew I could find and copy the word from one of the letters in the tray.

I typed something like this:

Dear…

Patrick is to have no more milk at break times.

Yors sincerely…

I concentrated so much on spelling 'sincerely' correctly that I missed out the 'u' in 'Yours'!

I folded the note up (not very neatly) and gave it to a member of staff the next day. She read the note standing in front of me and then asked, "Did your Mum write this or did you write it?" I couldn't lie. But I explained why and only drank cold milk from then on!

After school every day Mum and I went to meet Clare at the bus stop. I rode my big green tricycle along the seafront promenade there and back – a distance of about one mile. I sometimes got saddle sore!

Also while we were living in the seafront flat, we rented a VHS video recorder from the TV and video rental shop around the corner. It was the first video recorder we ever had and it came with a remote control. Well, it was actually a control with a long lead, which plugged into the video machine! The shop had a small selection of films to rent on video, including *The Cannonball Run*. Clare and I felt we hadn't seen the movie enough so we rented it a few times!

Southern Sound was something else I really enjoyed and they were running a charity appeal at the time. I kept hearing on the radio they were inviting people to go to their studios in Portslade (near Brighton), and donate non-perishable food for their 'food mountain'.

I really wanted to go and see the studios so, one evening, after school, we went and donated a few tins of food. I remember walking into the reception area, with my rollator, and seeing all of the black and white photos on the walls of each radio presenter. We also got to look through the window of one of the studios. I felt it was somewhere magical.

The person who greeted us asked me if I would like a mention on the radio.

"Yes please!" I replied excitedly. The guy wrote down my name and I asked, "Please could I have a mention tomorrow morning at 8.30 am because I'll be in my taxi on my way to school then."

The next day on the way to school, with Southern Sound on the radio, I said, "I'm going to get a mention on the radio!"

Tiny kept saying, "No you're not...!"

I kept saying, "Yes I am!"

After we heard the news at 8.30 am, Chris Copsey, the breakfast show presenter, said, "I must say hello and thank you to Patrick, who came into Southern Sound with some food yesterday and added it to our food mountain. Patrick, you're a megastar!"

Hearing that at ten years old was very exciting.

Not long after that I had the following conversation with Mum:

Me: "When I'm older I want to work in radio."

Mum: "I don't think you'll be able to do it as a full-time job. Maybe it's something you could do at the weekends."

We didn't live in the second floor flat for very long – only one or two months – before renting a three bedroom, semi-detached house in Feversham Close, on Shoreham Beach. The bedrooms and bathroom were upstairs so I had to keep walking up and down stairs for a bit longer!

It took over seven months to get the squatters evicted from Liz and John's house. Liz came back from Hong Kong twice to attend two court cases.

I got a new taxi driver – well, two of them – husband and wife, Mervin and Karen. They were nice people and we invited them over for dinner. They each drove a blue Lada and either one of them would pick me up to and from school. Karen had a Marvin Gaye tape with 'It Takes Two' and 'The Onion Song' on it, which developed my liking of Motown music.

In September 1984, Clare started at Steyning Grammar School (six miles north of Shoreham). This worked out well because Mandy and George had two grandsons, in Shoreham, who went to Steyning Grammar. George drove them to school every day and Mum shared the school run with him when Clare started at Steyning. George took Clare and his grandsons in the mornings and Mum picked them up every afternoon.

Once a week at Steyning, Clare and George's grandsons had after school activities. This meant that I would have arrived home from school before Mum and Clare did. At first, I stayed at Matthew Atwater's house (which was around the corner from us) for a while, until Mum came to get me. After a few weeks, Melvin and Karen dropped me off at home. (I thought about having house parties but I only had about twenty minutes before Mum and Clare arrived home!)

It was while we were living in Feversham Close that Mum bought me an Acorn Electron computer. She purchased it on finance, from Dixons, which had a high APR. We bought a cheap second-hand TV to go with it and set the computer up upstairs in my bedroom.

I remember the computer came with a brown cassette player and the volume had to be set at 2.5 in order for the games to load property! I had two games. Outrun – a car game, and Croaker – where you had to get five frogs (one at a time), across a busy motorway and then across a river, by jumping on a series of logs. Each game used to take about ten minutes to load, during which time the screen counted up in hexadecimal numbers.

The computer also provided me with my introduction to BASIC programming. I'm sure guys my age remember writing something like this!

10 Print "Hello, I'm Patrick!"

20 Goto 10

I learnt a fair bit from the manual which came with the computer and from a book called something like *101 Games for the Acorn Electron.*

I used to spend ages typing in lines of code from that book, only to find that most of the programmes didn't run! However, it was good fun sussing out what the problems were and making the programmes work. I learnt a lot by doing so. My Acorn Electron served me well.

My walking was going well too. It wasn't that long (a month or two), before I ditched my rollator and progressed onto using two walking sticks, which had four little legs on each stick (I think they are called quad sticks).

My rollator was too big and heavy – and no good with confined spaces! Once I started walking with my sticks I found I had to re-train my brain a bit. When I sensed I was starting to lose my balance, pulling on my sticks didn't help the situation (unlike my rollator, my sticks weren't a big and heavy object). Instead I had to learn to push down on my sticks to regain my balance.

In August 1984, Clare and I went to stay with Dad. We flew from Gatwick to Brussels and it was the first time Clare and I travelled on a plane unaccompanied. It was something we soon got accustomed to because we used to go and stay with Dad every school holiday. Normally, Clare and I went together but sometimes one of us went to see Dad on our own. It was easy because we/I always got assistance at the airport.

I have done a lot of travelling, and have been to many places in the world, on my own. Doing so has never worried me. I see it as an adventure!

It felt very strange staying in our old house in Belgium. I was still a bit emotionally attached to it because it felt like Dad, Yvonne and Juliet had invaded our old home. They had put new soft carpet upstairs, on the stairs and in the lounge (and maybe in the playroom – I don't remember!). A whole new kitchen had been installed. The cheap kitchen cupboards, which Mum used to moan about not opening and closing properly, had been replaced.

For some reason, Yvonne had repainted my old blue bedroom white. I didn't understand why she had done so, as it wasn't being used (Juliet had Clare's old room), and it upset me a bit. All there was in it was my old bed and an ironing board.

It was nice seeing Dad but he was at work most days. Hence, we were with Yvonne most of the time. It frustrated me because Clare and I had come to see Dad. Yvonne and I didn't get on well, especially when I was young. She disciplined me harshly and really made me cry the first time Clare and I went over to see Dad. It seemed like Yvonne wanted to exert her authority over me and was really strict. I didn't think she had the right to do so because she wasn't my mother.

Dad did have a few days off work while we were there. I remember getting up early and watching the previous day's highlights of the Olympics in Los Angles on TV. Also, I was able to drive the lawnmower around the garden again and I now knew how to stop it!

The subsequent times we went to see Dad, while he was still living in Belgium, we flew to Maastricht, as it's closer to Liege than Brussels is.

Back in England, we moved into Liz and John's house on 19th November 1984 (two days before my eleventh Birthday). After waiting for more than seven months for the squatters to get their marching orders, it was nice to finally move into the house. I had one of the downstairs bedrooms at the back of the house so I no longer needed to walk up and down stairs!

However, it took me a few days to master how to walk up the front doorstep. It was quite a high step and unlike stairs, there was no banister or wall to lean on.

I have always been able to get anywhere I want to go to in life. It's all due to my mindset, determination and experience.

I had an eleventh birthday party at McDonald's. Lots of friends from school came. Afterwards, we all went across the road to the cinema and saw the film *Ghostbusters*. It was a good cinema because it was accessible for my friends in wheelchairs.

As I said in Chapter One, I have been through some dark and difficult times so far in life (and have overcome them all). What you're about to read about is the most personal thing in *Stairs For Breakfast*.

When I first had the idea of writing a book about me in November 2010, I spent two and a half years thinking about what to put in it, before I started to write the book.

At first, I decided not to include what I'm about to tell you because it is incredibly personal. However, as I continued to think about the book I realised that if I left this part out, most of the rest of my book wouldn't make much sense. What I am about to disclose has dramatically affected my life.

I decided, therefore, that it had to be included. I then thought: *How on earth do I describe what happened?* Needless to say, I have thought a lot about this section of the book over the last two and a half years.

I didn't speak to anyone about what happened in 1984 until I was twenty-six (in 2000). It was only then that I began to realise how, and why, the relationship occurred. Ironically, it wasn't until I got into property investment much later on and started making videos of my property journey – and I saw myself on camera – that I completely understood. The fact that I can now talk about it so candidly means it doesn't matter to me anymore.

* * * *

At middle school I had another friend called Nathan, who was also ten years old. He didn't appear to be disabled and I don't know what his condition was. Nathan was attached to Pebbles but had all of his lessons in the main school.

For many years after (until 2000, when I discovered why it had occurred), I classed the friendship I had had with him as "inappropriate". Nathan often stayed overnight at my house (every one to two weeks) and we slept in the same bed. Fortunately, we didn't know what sex was.

I did go to Nathan's house a few times after school, but I don't remember ever staying the night there. His family used to eat dinner (or tea) at 4.30 pm in the afternoon!

I don't remember exactly when our friendship started and ended, but I think it lasted six to eight months. Nathan started to stay over when we lived at Feversham Close and I guesstimate the friendship ended in January 1985. Once we moved to Feversham Close, Nathan and I went to school in the same taxi.

However, I do remember how it started and ended. It began while I was walking around the playground with my rollator when Nathan got me to go in the tent (on the grass area) with him. (Zoe also got me to go into the tent with her, where she showed me her vagina.)

My advice to schools is: do not put a tent in the playground because you do not know what goes on in there. I didn't go to school wanting to start an inappropriate relationship with a boy (nor did I wish to see Zoe's vagina).

Now that I understand that experimentation and sexual play is a normal part of childhood development, I am at peace about the relationship I had with Nathan. However, as a ten or eleven-year-old boy, I wasn't happy about it because I didn't instigate the relationship and because I didn't understand what was going on. I thought it was wrong.

The property we lived in at Fevesham Close wasn't a big house. The three bedrooms upstairs were all next to one another.

Mum and Clare knew what was going on because they saw Nathan and I kissing and hugging each other.

In December, Nathan gave me a Christmas card. I remember standing near the kitchen bin, when Mum caught me as I was about to tear the card up into little pieces and bury it in the bin.

"What are you doing?" Mum asked. She took the card out of my hand and read out loud, "To Patrick, Love Nathan," and then asked, "What's wrong with that?"

The relationship had affected my confidence and I was speechless – I didn't know what to say.

However, it was the following incident that has caused me a number of emotional and psychological problems, over so many years.

For some reason Nathan was in hospital for a few days, where Mum and I went to visit him. At the time, Mum was still carrying me and pushing me around in my buggy when we went out somewhere, as I was only walking short distances.

Nathan was lying on the hospital bed and I was sitting on the edge of it. Mum picked me up, as we were about to leave the hospital, when the following was said and done:

Mum: (holding me in her arms) "Why don't you kiss each other goodbye?"

Me: "No, I don't want to." I brushed my hand from right to left to form a metaphorical barrier.

Mum: (in a jovial voice) "Go on... I won't look!"

Nathan: "Go on...!"

Mum then held me towards Nathan and he kissed me. I clearly said, "No, I don't want to," beforehand.

I was so upset, shocked and angry by the incident in the hospital – and by what I felt, at the time, was an inappropriate relationship with Nathan.

However, I still felt very dependent on Mum, and therefore, I didn't know how to express my feelings to her. Hence, I didn't say anything to her about it. I kept all my feelings bottled up – and we have never discussed Nathan.

I wasn't in the habit of kissing people. Other than my family, the only other person I had kissed was Dominique on our way to and from school in Belgium. I knew I wasn't gay, but because Mum and Clare witnessed Nathan and I together, I was convinced that they thought I was gay.

Writing about it today – being much older and knowing what I now know about childhood development and human behaviour, I can see why the friendship with Nathan started. I was a shy new boy at school and, walking with my rollator, may have appeared to be a very vulnerable person.

In my mind, I don't think I'm disabled – but seeing myself on video, I appear to be very disabled – and it's how most people see me. Appearances can be deceptive.

At the time of my relationship with Nathan, I thought it was wrong and that Mum should have stopped it. However now, I think Mum saw it as a harmless friendship. I love my mum and she was the one who, pretty much single-handedly, brought me (and Clare) up. If it wasn't for her, I may not have turned out to be such an achiever.

I also think my relationship with Mum became so turbulent partly because we never discussed my friendship with Nathan.

Back at school, soon after the hospital incident, I ended my friendship with Nathan by scratching his face quite badly. I scratched his face severely enough that I was petrified of going to school the next day. I thought his mum was going to be there complaining about what I had done to her son's face. (A few months later I refused to sign Nathan's birthday card, as it was being passed around Pebbles.)

Shortly after I ended my friendship with Nathan, I suffered the most embarrassing moment in my life.

Sitting in my class one afternoon, I suddenly weed myself. I remember the sound the urine made as it splashed onto the floor – and then everybody turning around and looking at me. I just wanted the world to open up and swallow me. My teacher asked a member of my class to go to get the janitor and a member of staff from Pebbles.

I don't remember if I weed myself because someone made me laugh, which occasionally happened when I was younger (is that where the phrase 'I peed myself laughing' comes from?). Or whether it was because I was anxious and not looking forward to the next three days.

My class was going on a three day trip to London to visit the Science Museum, the Natural History Museum and Madame Tussauds. My teacher had arranged for Mum to come on the trip so she could push me in my wheelchair and look after me.

The next morning as I walked onto the coach, with Mum behind me, all my friends were asking me whether I was okay and if I needed to go to the toilet. I felt extremely embarrassed and unhappy. It wasn't an enjoyable three days for me because I really resented Mum being there. None of the other kids had their mum there and I felt she didn't understand me anymore.

Another odd thing happened in the first three months of 1985 when I developed a fear of abandonment. It was the same fear I once felt in Belgium, when I waited in the car while Mum went into a shop for such a long time, I thought something had happened to her and she wasn't going to come back. However, the fear I now had felt much stronger.

On Wednesdays, Mum started an evening class in Worthing, and Clare and I stayed at home alone. We always watched *Dallas* on TV, which ended at 9.00 pm – the same time that Mum's class finished. By 9.30 pm I would start worrying that Mum had been raped or murdered, walking the dark, mean streets of Worthing(!).

I got myself into such a severe state of panic and crying that Clare could not stop me from crawling (which was faster than walking), out of the house and onto the pavement, from where I could see cars coming up the road, waiting for Mum.

It was such a relief when she got home every week. Mum was always furious with me. Her way of dealing with the situation was by shouting at me and telling me not to be so stupid. Which didn't help at all.

I had a few weeks of therapy for my fear of abandonment, which slowly dissipated and I overcame it within six to twelve months.

Writing about it (my fear of abandonment), now is strange. On the one hand it makes me feel embarrassed. One the other hand I find it funny because I'm happier not knowing where my mum is in the world.

Since deciding to detach myself from my family in 2011, I've achieved so much and am a lot happier, without the stress and pressure that Mum was causing me. My wish for Mum is that she becomes at peace with herself and other people.

I was no longer a happy boy, without a care in life. I felt ashamed. Although I didn't understand why my friendship with Nathan had happened, I felt partly responsible for it because I went along with it. It turned me into an unhappy person and I learnt to live with it. Over the years I got to thinking it was something odd that had happened.

It affected my confidence in life. No longer did I want to bring any of my friends home because I thought Mum would think that I wanted to sleep with them. At school, I was my normal self around my friends. At home I felt embarrassed mentioning my friends. On the occasions when I was out somewhere with Mum or Clare and we bumped into any of my friends, I quickly became red-faced with embarrassment.

Another thing that developed was my nervous cough – and it's something I still do sometimes today. The more nervous I feel the louder I cough.

Watching TV with Mum or Clare became uncomfortable. My body involuntarily jumped at scenes of a sexual or intimate nature or on hearing words such as 'sex', 'gay', 'kiss' or 'love'. It felt horrible. Over the years, I tried so hard not to react but there was nothing I could do to stop myself jumping – so I just accepted it. Ironically, it perpetuated Mum and Clare's belief that I was gay.

I have never had the confidence to say to Mum or Clare, "I know you think I'm gay, but I am not."

My mum has always been (or tried to be), very domineering and controlling with me and Clare. Over the years following my friendship with Nathan, my relationship with Mum changed. No longer was I prepared to do everything she said. It triggered a battle of power and control. Our relationship became increasingly more turbulent as I got older.

In the summer of 1985, I left middle school and I don't know which school Nathan went on to.

At the beginning of this piece of the book, I alluded to being twenty-six-years-old before gaining an understanding of why my relationship with Nathan occurred. All I will say for now is everything is in this book. Keep on reading!

* * * *

Soon after we moved into Liz and John's house in November 1984 I joined the 3rd Shoreham Sea Scouts. I received a Hobbies & Interests badge for my postcard collection, which I had started when we lived in Belgium.

The house needed some odd jobs doing to it so Mandy and George (who we stayed with when we moved back to England), recommended a handyman called Eric, who lived down the road with his wife and two kids. Eric was a good guy and would often come to do odd jobs for us around the house. I would help him by passing him tools from his knackered old tool bag, when he was up the ladder. Eric became a family friend and popped in for a coffee now and again.

At Christmas, Nan and Grandad came to stay with us. It was good to see them because it was the first time that they came to stay with us since we moved back to England.

They now tended to come by train and stay with us for a week, every five or six weeks. Well, I say they – more often than not, Nan came on her own because Grandad preferred to stay at home in London on his own. And I think Nan liked having a break from Grandad!

By the beginning of 1985 my walking was improving and I was managing to walk further and further distances. Sometime in the first quarter of 1985 I ditched my quad sticks in favour of walking sticks with three legs (in my mind, they should be called tri-sticks! Why aren't they?).

I had also pretty much outgrown my buggy. Therefore, it was around this time that I got a Bromakin Spinner – a lightweight, blue wheelchair. It was really good because it meant I could now go somewhere on my own. At the weekends I often went to the shops at the end of our road (about a quarter of a mile away). I tended to go to the newsagents and to the café for a cappuccino and cake. It was nice to go out with Mum or Clare in my wheelchair – rather than in my buggy – because it made me feel more grown up and in control.

My wheelchair had anti-tip bars to prevent me from doing too much of a wheelie – tipping backwards and smashing my head on the ground! Also, on the back of the wheelchair was a holder for my sticks. This enabled me to also walk places when I went out, for example, if a shop had steps into it I could leave my wheelchair outside and walk into the shop. Once I built up more stamina pushing myself in my wheelchair I went further afield. I could go across the footbridge and into Shoreham town (I was more like twelve-years- old when I did this). I became confident crossing main roads and getting to wherever I wanted to go.

Although my lightweight wheelchair was easier for me to push than my DHSS wheelchair at school, it still required a lot of effort and energy, due to my poor coordination.

When I used to push myself to the shops along the road we lived in, I used the pavement on both sides of the road, depending on whether I was on my way out or coming home. It was a lot easier to go along the pavement, where the gradient of the pavement sloped into the road (eg where the road was on my left). This enabled me to use my left hand to do all (most) of the pushing, whilst holding the palm of my right hand against the rim of the right wheel, keeping the wheelchair going in a straight line.

Outside, there are very few totally flat surfaces. Wheelchairs are also hard to push on carpets. Surfaces at airports are the easiest to push myself in my wheelchair because the ground is flat and gives little friction. Obviously, it's easy going downhill in a wheelchair, whilst going up any kind of hill or bump is difficult.

I rarely use my wheelchair these days. I stopped using it when I learnt to drive (when I was seventeen). Today, I drive my car to wherever I'm going and walk the rest of the way. The only time I use my wheelchair now is when I go on holiday. The rest of the time, it lives in the boot of my car. I really don't like using my wheelchair. I'll explain why later in this book.

In April/May 1985 John (my uncle), came back from Hong Kong for a few weeks on business and he stayed with us. Never will I forget staying up past midnight with John one night, watching the final of the snooker world championship, between Steve Davies and Dennis Taylor. The game went to the deciding frame and both players kept failing to pot the final black ball. This is what started me liking to watch snooker.

John worked for a travel magazine in Hong Kong and he had access to cheap flights and holidays. Normally, Liz, John and my three cousins came back to England during the summer. However, Liz and John decided to treat us all to a two week holiday in Thailand that summer – and then Mum, Clare and I would go back to Hong Kong and stay with them in their apartment for another two weeks. It sounded like an exciting holiday.

My walking with tri-sticks was going well – but I knew I could do better. I wanted to walk with crutches. I saw crutches as being the Rolls Royce of walking sticks because, unlike my quad and tri-sticks, crutches didn't remain upright on their own. Hence, I set myself a goal; to be walking with crutches by the time we went on holiday to Thailand and Hong Kong in July.

By May, I wasn't enjoying Sea Scouts anymore. Socially, my confidence was low, I felt withdrawn and I didn't feel I could achieve much there. Sea scouting involved doing a lot of physical activities, like building rafts out of bits of wood. I would just sit in the old DHSS wheelchair they had there and watch everyone else doing things. I felt that I was useless when I was there, so I decided to leave the Sea Scouts.

In July, Martin, Matthew Atwater, Richard Smith and I, left middle school to start at our secondary school in September.

Liz and my cousin Becky came to England for a couple of weeks before our summer holiday. Then Clare and Becky flew to Hong Kong a week before Liz, Mum and I flew to Bangkok. Our holiday started well because John had managed to blag business class tickets for us on Thai Airways, who provided an excellent journey.

The whole family met in Bangkok. There were eight of us and we stayed in a brand new four star hotel for three days. I remember riding around in a tuk-tuk (a motorbike-taxi) in Bangkok.

We then hired a small minibus and drove to Hua Hin. The hotel we stayed at in Hua Hin had an outdoor swimming pool, which was surrounded by little bedroom balconies. While we were staying there, it wasn't uncommon for people to jump off one of the second floor balconies, into the swimming pool. Damian was doing it, Keith was doing it – and I think Clare and Becky had a go. Of course I wanted to do it too!

The thought of jumping into the pool from the second floor balcony scared me but the fear I felt was overtaken by the thrill and anticipation of doing the jump. I wanted to do it with my armbands on but Mum wouldn't let me wear them, as she said it would ruin the photograph she was going to take.

I jumped off the balcony with John and Keith on either side of me. As we were in mid-air, I felt John let go of my arm so I quickly grabbed hold of his! After we splashed into the pool, I didn't resurface for a few seconds – but John grabbed me – and I was fine! (I think because I was a lot lighter than John and Keith, I didn't bounce as much as they did!)

It was one of those things I had to do in life. And somewhere, there's a mid-air photo of me, John and Keith jumping into the pool. I think it's in an old suitcase of photos that either Clare or Mum has.

Keith was the only person who jumped into the pool from a third floor balcony.

After we had stayed in Hua Hin for a week or so, we went to Pattaya for the remainder of our holiday in Thailand. In Pattaya, Toyota pickups are used as taxis!

It was either in Hua Hin or Pattaya where we went parasailing over the Thai sea (parasailing, over the sea, is where you're towed by a speed boat, while attached to a parachute. The combination of these two things makes you go high up in the sky!).

I went up with one of the instructors behind me. It was great fun. We took off from the sandy beach. I seem to remember the instructor lifted me up, and took a few steps forwards to get airborne. Parasailing isn't the most exhilarating thing I've ever done – but it's up there!

While in Thailand I collected a number of cuts on my legs, from crawling in and out of swimming pools. By the time we got to Hong Kong my cuts had become infected so I went to see a doctor, with Liz and Mum. The doctor gave me some antibiotics and advised Mum to bathe my legs with warm salty water.

Back at Liz and John's apartment that evening, Mum made some warm salty water in a plastic jug and slowly poured it over my wounds. When she had poured all of the water over my legs Mum noticed there was some undissolved salt left in the jug. Without thinking, she poured the undissolved salt onto one of my wounds. I have never screamed so loudly in my life.

Despite that little mishap, Honkers was good fun. I bought a little radio alarm clock, which also had a miniature black and white TV. It was nice spending time with my cousins and the food was good. I developed a real liking for Vita lemon tea, which is best drank in hot weather (it doesn't taste so good in the UK when it's windy and raining!).

I also learnt some Cantonese while in Hong Kong. I can count up to 100 (if you can count up to ten in Cantonese, you can count up to 100) and, "Hello, how are you?" which sounds something like, 'Josan, lay-ho-ma'.

It was a very good summer holiday. Mum, Clare and I flew back to England in business class as well!

Being a well-travelled person, it's not the only time I've flown business class or been to Thailand. Having just written about it makes me want to go back to Thailand now!

Oh yes – I started walking with crutches in June 1985.

In April 1984, I went from crawling and not being able to walk (apart from up and down stairs), to walking with a rollator, onto quad sticks, onto tri-sticks, and then walking with crutches – within fifteen months. I'm proud with this achievement.

Chapter 4

I n August 1985, a few weeks before I started at secondary school, we received a letter informing us that I was going to be picked up at 7.45 am every morning and taken to school by minibus. It came as a shock that I was going to be picked up so early. I wasn't happy about it, but there was nothing I could do about it.

During my three years at secondary school, I went to school in the same minibus, with some of my disabled friends that I had been at middle school with (including Martin, Matthew, Richard and Justin). Six out of the eight kids on the bus were in wheelchairs, and used the tailgate lift to get on and off the minibus. I sat in a normal seat and walked on and off via the front door.

The minibus was 'manned' by Donald and Enid (who sound like a married couple but they just worked together!) Donald, in his sixties, drove the bus and operated the wheelchair lift at the back of the vehicle. Enid, in her forties or fifties, took people on or off the bus and strapped everyone's wheelchair to the floor.

Leaving at 7.45 am and getting home at 4.45 pm, my day felt quite long. It took about 50 minutes to get to school, as I was the second person picked up in the morning, and the last one to be dropped home in the afternoon. Emily was the first person to be collected in the morning – then after me were Matthew and Martin respectively. Because we four lived the furthest from school, we were the core people on the bus over the three years.

Don and Enid were nice people. Don often liked to have a few cigarette puffs when he got off the bus to operate the lift.

Initially, attending secondary school excited me a bit. Similar to my previous school, it had a unit – called Barley – for disabled kids. I had some lessons in the main school and some in Barley.

The first thing I thought about my new school was the uniform was a bit stupid! It included a dark yellow shirt. I ask you, why would anyone think that a dark yellow shirt would be appealing to eleven to eighteen-year-old kids?

My second impression was that Miss Monroe, the head of Barley, was a bit too overbearing! She was in her late thirties, not very tall, with short dark hair, steely blue eyes and wore thick round glasses. Oh, and she was a nun and lived in a convent!

It didn't take me long to settle in at my new school and I made friends, both in Barley and in the main school. The two disabled people who spring to mind are Richard Buss and Fergus. Richard Buss had MD and we were in the same tutor group together (in the main school).

Fergus didn't appear to be disabled and was quite a loud person. He was always running round everywhere and willing to help everyone. At break times, in Barley, Fergus and another boy (Giles) had a music system from somewhere and were often playing music. They always seemed to have the latest seven inch chart records.

Fergus and I are still friends today – and I'm sure we'll still be friends when we're eighty. Well, I'll be eighty and he'll be eighty-two! Fergus is always happy and never has a bad word to say about anyone – not even traffic wardens!

In the main school I was friends with James, Curtis and Ricky. There was a girl in my tutor group whom I got the impression liked me. She had long brown hair and I think her name was Rachel. I spoke with her sometimes, but I only had the confidence to ask how she was.

I have always liked helping people. At school I regularly helped my friends with MD by getting something out of their bag for them or helping them to have a drink, by holding a cup whilst they drank from it using a straw. I was pleased to help them (and others); it's something that I did without thinking.

Martin and Justin were still quite strong at the time. Richard Smith, Richard Buss and Matthew Atwater were weaker and needed more help. I didn't help Matthew a great deal because he used to moan a lot, which meant other people helped him. Both of the Richards were more easy-going.

Matthew was extremely mature and bright for his age – he knew his life was going to be short. I felt extremely sorry for Matthew – and for everyone I knew with MD.

It makes me feel grateful having CP.

I was never naughty at secondary school but it's fair to say that I was unruly. I've never been someone to conform easily to something I don't agree with. I was rather loud and outspoken at school - I was often having a laugh and a joke and larking around with people. Because I was reserved at home, I think I made up for it at school.

Monroe obviously didn't appreciate my behaviour much because she frequently hauled me into her office, sometimes along with Martin.

Going into Monroe's office always followed the same process. It would start with her staring, silently, at me through her thick glasses for about a minute. It was slightly intimidating at first but then I thought she wanted a staring contest! Then came her rambling on at me about something that I had said or done. I thought it was pathetic. She only ever had a go at me because I was outspoken and because I did things that other kids didn't do. Monroe once called me into her office because I had had my packed lunch in the main school (rather than in Barley).

As I mentioned in the previous chapter I was in a class with kids a year younger than me. When I started at secondary school I was put in classes for my age group. Effectively, I skipped a school year.

The only books (apart from Ladybird ones) I had read up to that point were:

- *Jonathan Livingston Seagull*
- One book of *Tales of the Unexpected* by Roald Dahl

The Complete Fawlty Towers (my favourite TV programme and which I knew every line of, before reading the book).

I can only remember my time at secondary school as a whole and don't remember each year individually. I did so many subjects over the three years. Here's my synopsis of what I thought about each one.

Main school classes:

Art

I've never been an arty person, and with my wobbly handwriting, art was the most pointless subject I ever did. It would be akin to a blind person having driving lessons.

History

I found history boring and tedious. Being a modern type of guy, I wasn't interested in what happened hundreds and thousands of years ago.

I came a bit unstuck recently when someone mentioned William Wallace to me. I was like, "William who...? Never heard of him." It was a little embarrassing.

Geography

Learning about different countries and cultures has always interested me. However, the geography I did at school was more along the lines of how lakes and rivers are formed and what minerals are in the ground. I found geography similar to my history lessons.

I learnt more about countries around the world from the computer game I had on my Acorn Electron, where you had to name capital cities.

RE

I have always respected people's religious beliefs and always been of the opinion that you shouldn't force religion onto people. (At school in Belgium we were given the choice to do RE or not.)

In my RE classes, using my Brother typewriter, I just plagiarised the smallest paragraph from the book or hand-out we were using on the day.

Biology

I don't remember learning much about the human body in biology. I've never been very good when it comes to blood and guts (or needles) and I don't know much about how the body works. All I know is that it does (and cuts and bruises mend themselves).

The biology I did at school was mostly to do with plants and insects – which didn't float my boat much.

Chemistry

I'm no scientist. But I enjoyed mixing up chemicals and playing with Bunsen burners! Especially the experiments where you were advised to put on plastic glasses – because it normally meant that some sort of bang or explosion was about to occur!

Physics

I liked physics but all I remember learning is that the opposite ends of two magnets stick together.

In biology, chemistry and physics I had one of the Barley classroom assistants with me to help me do the experiments (and to ensure I didn't set the place on fire). I felt I didn't need any help and would have preferred to do the experiments with my classmates. I sat at front of the class with my assistant, and the rest of the class sat behind us. I felt slightly segregated, which I didn't like much.

French

There wasn't a lot of point in me doing French. I sat back and enjoyed the class. The teacher often asked me if what he was teaching the class was correct.

German

I only did German for a term. Learning to speak it was okay but I was poor at reading and writing it. I learnt to count to twenty and to say, "Guten tag, mein name ist Patrick, ich bin dreizehn jahre alt und ich lebe in Shoreham." (I find it easier to write these days – using Google Translator!)

Barley classes:

Cookery

I did cookery one afternoon a week, where I made a few nice cakes and puddings. However, I didn't learn anything in cookery to help me later on in life, when it came to cooking and eating healthily every day. I taught myself that.

Horse riding

On Tuesday afternoons Donald and Enid took five or six of us horse riding.

We rode the same horse every week. I had a knackered old grey horse called Blue, which didn't go very fast. I had to wear a belt around my tummy (as did everyone else) which had handles on it. I had one person holding onto me and another person leading my horse, using a rope which was attached to the bit in its mouth. All we did was walk slowly round the stable school in circles. It was boring, boring, boring. In the summer we sometimes went outside, walking along a narrow country path – which still wasn't much fun. However, sitting on a horse gave my abductor muscles quite a good stretch.

My idea of horse riding was to go galloping off somewhere!

IT

I remember having lessons in the Barley computer room but I don't remember doing anything on the computers – apart from playing Chuckie Egg sometimes at lunchtime.

Swimming

I went swimming once a week in the Barley hydrotherapy pool. Swimming in such warm water was really nice. The air around the pool was extremely hot and stuffy and the time it took me getting changed was uncomfortable. I had to have help getting my shoes and socks on/off because the bench in the changing room was too high and narrow to do so myself.

Sex education

This consisted of Monroe unwrapping a condom one lunchtime and showing it to us. Very appetising! (I love the irony of a nun unwrapping a condom.)

The more astute of you reading this may have noticed that I haven't included the core subjects; Maths and English.

Upon starting at secondary school, I was put in the top Maths class in my year. There were thirty-five kids in the class and the academic year seemed to start with a trigonometry test, which for some reason I handwrote the answers to. It was embarrassing because I only answered this one question correctly 'What is a three-sided shape called?' I hadn't done any trigonometry before (I think it must have been taught in the school year that I had just skipped). Therefore, I had Maths lessons in Barley with three deaf kids. I found that Maths too basic (I only remember doing percentages).

While writing this part of the book for the last few days, I've been trying to recall what English lessons I had. I find it astonishing that I can remember doing an array of different subjects but I don't remember having any English lessons.

I think I had English lessons with Mrs Brown (deputy head of Barley). The only reason I think I did is because, in 1986, I went through a one or two month phase of reading the *Today* newspaper. We had it delivered at home in the mornings and I took it to school every day. I remember Mrs Brown letting me read it during class time because she said it was grown up of me do to so.

I have written the synopsis of my lessons at school from a slightly humorous angle. However, the serious point of it is far more important and relevant.

The other reason I was so boisterous at school was because I wasn't being mentally stimulated. It wasn't that I didn't want to learn. I've always been interested in learning new things. I wasn't put in the right classes.

If I wasn't up to the top Maths class for my year, why on earth wasn't I put into the class below it? I needed to learn algebra and trigonometry. Why didn't I have proper English lessons in the three years I was at secondary school? As I'm writing this now, I'm thinking, *why didn't I kick up a fuss about not having proper Maths and English?* The answer to that is I was eleven, twelve, thirteen and fourteen-years-old.

I think Monroe was totally irresponsible not to see what the problem was. She was the head of Barley and she knew that I was intelligent. Rather than telling me off in her office every five minutes, Monroe should have put me in the appropriate classes. It wasn't rocket science. Mum saw the problem so why didn't Monroe?

I don't remember ever being given any books to read at school or much homework. It seemed to me that they thought I had a hard enough life and long day at school.

The truth is – had I been taught proper English and Maths at secondary school Mum wouldn't have carted me off to boarding school. Mum did absolutely the right thing.

Another thing which seemed to flummox Monroe was when I wanted to go to the local fish and chip shop at lunchtime with James and a few other mates. Monroe's stance was that I needed to get my mum's written permission first. Which I did. Nevertheless, I felt it was ridiculous not having equal rights as my able-bodied friends.

I only use my wheelchair when somewhere is too far for me to walk to. Therefore at school, I used my wheelchair in the main school but walked in Barley.

One Christmastime at school I was one of the boys who queued up to kiss Emily under the mistletoe. It was worth the wait!

Donald drove the minibus ten minutes faster on the way to school than on the way home. He didn't want to arrive late at school in the mornings because he was scared of Monroe. Equally, it seemed to me, he didn't want to arrive home too early in the afternoons because he didn't get on so well with his wife!

Away from school in autumn 1985, our Toyota Corona was dying. It was using as much oil as petrol. Therefore Mum purchased, through the Motability scheme, a new silver grey Vauxhall Astra. It was nice not to be seen in that Belgium-Japanese rust-bucket anymore!

I've got a good memory for car number plates, as well as for numbers, because I can still remember our Belgian number plate.

My walking was going well and I was managing to walk further and further distances. However, I was becoming quite asthmatic so Mum took me to see Alison Smith, our family GP, who prescribed me an inhaler.

We had been to see Alison before, shortly after we moved back to England. I would like to give you a picture of what Alison looked like in the mid-eighties. She looked a bit like the lady who plays the doctor, in the white coat and glasses, in Marvin Gaye's 'Sexual Healing' video. Even as a ten and eleven-year-old boy I thought Alison was hot!

Alison was an excellent doctor, who remained my GP until she retired at the end of 2012.

Up until the time we moved into Liz and John's house, most of our furniture from Belgium was in storage, including the Phillips television we had had for years. When I was twelve, the TV remote control broke. The TV itself was fine. I thought *I must be able to get a new remote control for it.*

I got the phone number for the Phillips UK head office from directory enquiries, phoned them and explained the problem. The lady I spoke to gave me the name and address of the guy I needed to write to. I typed and sent a letter, giving the model number of the TV. Shortly after, I received a package with a letter saying 'This remote control might not work. Let me know if it doesn't and I'll send you a different one'. The remote control didn't work so I phoned the guy up and he sent me another one which did work. I phoned him again, when I received the second remote control, to thank him very much for his help. It was an easy job well done. The TV (and remote control) lasted another ten years.

Something I haven't mentioned yet in this book is my speech, which has been affected by my CP. Not everyone with CP has problems with speech. It depends on the brain damage caused at birth, by the lack of oxygen and the severity of the disability.

It's unfortunate that my speech has been affected because, had it not have been, it would have made my life much easier.

When I talk, the voice I hear sounds perfectly normal. However, when I hear myself on tape or video I sound so disabled. I know everyone thinks they sound different on tape but I find it strange hearing such a big discrepancy in my voice.

Speaking on the phone is something I've always been confident at doing. Well, 99% of the time. People have often said that I speak more clearly on the phone than I do in person. However, I become self-conscious about my voice and nervous speaking to someone, on the phone, who I haven't spoken to before – and who I feel I need to impress.

The reason is simple. When I meet someone in person, they can clearly see that I'm disabled. On the phone, they can't see me.

For example, I would get nervous phoning someone about a job interview. For the first few seconds of the call, until the other person knows who I am and what I'm calling about, I would hyperventilate a bit and not have enough air to talk properly. It feels horrible.

I've got a couple of strategies to overcome it. First I do, what I think of as, a warm up call – call someone who doesn't make me feel nervous. Doing this relaxes me and makes me feel more confident. The second strategy, which relaxes me, is having some background music on when I make an important phone call.

It seems odd writing about it today because I overcame that fear a few years ago. Also I don't apply for jobs these days!

When I went out and about in my wheelchair when I was twelve-years-old, I started noticing something which I didn't like. People tended to talk down to me, as if I was stupid. I had to find a way overcome it. (I remember a kid at school asking me "Do all your family talk like you do?")

The woman who owned my local newsagents used to annoy me. She was a lady in her fifties who spoke in a soft voice and often asked me, "Would you like an ice cream?"

I always replied, "No thank you, I don't like ice cream." (When we lived in Belgium, I fell and broke one of my front teeth. This caused me to have sensitive teeth.)

I thought: *If I start talking to people and helping them they will see that I'm not an idiot.* So that's what I started doing – particularly at school. What happened really surprised me. As I began to help people they started to open up and warm to me. So I helped people more and more – and they got to know me. Also, people began to help me, without me even asking them for help! I didn't understand why at the time.

I believe in helping people as much as I can in life. I'll explain why later on in the book.

At home, doing her evening class in communications, Mum was always going on about body language and, specifically, how important it is to make eye-contact with people.

So I tried it myself, when I went out and about. I was amazed at how powerful it is. When I was out somewhere and I made eye-contact with a stranger, they would always ask me if they could help me.

This is what sparked my interest in human behaviour and psychology.

Eye-contact is something I use today. If I would like someone's help I just make eye-contact with them. It is so powerful. Conversely, when I don't want people to help me I don't look at them.

I have always been a perceptive and an intuitive person. Once I discovered the power of helping people and of eye-contact, I began to watch people's behaviour and body language – and to listen to what people were saying – more intently. I've learnt so much from doing so.

Back to when I was twelve, my bedroom wasn't that big. We had been to MFI a few times (does anyone remember the flat-pack furniture store MFI? Some people called it Made For Idiots!), and I had my eye on one of those melamine bunk beds – where the bed is on top and below it is a wardrobe, a desk area and a set of three drawers. The only issue was, it came with a piddly ladder (which attached to the front of the bed). The ladder wasn't any good for me because the rungs on it were too small. However, we measured the length of the bed to see if it would fit in my bedroom.

When we got home Mum measured the wall in my room. The bed would fit along the wall, leaving a little gap at the foot of the bed. I then had the idea that we could get handyman Eric to saw off the piece of melamine at the foot-end of the bed and we could get a normal domestic ladder, and wedge it (folded up) against the end of the bunk bed and the wall. So that's what we did!

I got it as a Christmas present. Clare and Eric put the bunk bed together (Clare has always been good at building flatpack furniture). And Eric sawed the border at the foot of the bed off. We bought a normal ladder, with a metal frame and wooden rungs. The top of the ladder rested against the bed, whilst the feet of the ladder were wedged against the skirting board of the facing wall. The ladder never moved.

At first I enjoyed the novelty of climbing up a ladder to get into bed! Then for the next three years I did it without thinking about it. Climbing the ladder was easy because I only had to climb up four rungs. I propped my crutches against the wall on my left and held onto both sides of the ladder to climb it.

In the mornings, I reversed myself out of bed and put my feet on the third rung of the ladder. My crutches were in easy reach when I got down it. In three years, I never fell down the ladder.

Something which Mum organised for me in 1986 was to go weight training one evening a week at Lewes Prison (sixteen miles east of Shoreham). Mum took me there every week. I was one of five disabled people who went weight training in the prison gym. Each of us got buddied-up with a prison inmate. I was good at bench-pressing weights. The inmates were nice people. I didn't have the nerve to ask my buddy why he was in prison. On arriving at, and leaving, the prison a security guard escorted us through a load of metal barrier-doors/gates, which felt really weird! Weight training was good fun and I did it for about six months. All of the other disabled people were adults.

Mum decided she wanted Clare and I to have nice straight teeth, which involved a series of trips to the dentist and orthodontist in 1986. Our dentist was good and a nice guy, unlike the orthodontist who didn't have many people-skills, and his practice was up a flight of stairs.

Clare got away with it lightly. She only had a retainer for her top teeth. I got the full metal works – aka tram-lines – with elastic bands, from top to bottom, on both sides inside my mouth. Some people at school called me Jaws!

My brace became problematic over the two years that I had it. Twice our dentist saw me, as an emergency on Sunday, when part of my brace became unstuck and an end of it was poking into my gum, making it bleed.

Clare had her first boyfriend (Joel) when she was fourteen. In the summer of 1986, Mum, Clare and I went on a cheap two-week package and self-catering holiday to Majorca with Joel, his mum and his sister – called Natasha.

It wasn't the best holiday I've ever been on. Monarch Airlines left my wheelchair in the jetty at Gatwick so I was without it for the first three days of the holiday. When we were reunited with my wheelchair, Mum took the anti-tip bars off of it, to make it easier to push me up and down the high Majorcan pavements.

I developed a bit of a holiday crush for Natasha (who was a year older than me). I wanted to let her know that I liked her but not being a confident person, it took me four days to pluck up the courage to tell her. One afternoon while playing on the beach with Natasha, I looked at my Casio digital watch. It was 14:27 and I decided that now was the right time to tell her – so I forced myself to say, "I fancy you." Natasha didn't respond. I thought maybe she did hear or understand me so I said again, "I fancy you," but she didn't react.

I was disappointed that Natasha didn't say anything but I felt good that I plucked up the courage to tell her.

A few days later while I was chasing Natasha around, in my wheelchair, on the veranda of our villa, I got a bit too excited, pressed down too much on the back wheels of my wheelchair, tipped myself backwards and cracked the back of my head on the tiled floor and spent two nights in a Majorcan hospital!

It taught me not to chase girls round Majorcan verandas without my anti-tip bars!

In September of 1986 my Grandpa died suddenly. He got up out of bed one Sunday morning and went to the bathroom, where he keeled over from a heart-attack.

It was a strange week; on the Monday I went to school as normal, knowing that Grandpa had died. On Tuesday Clare and I flew to Antwerp.

Clare and I were used to flying to Maastricht (to stay with dad) on a 100-seater plane, which we considered to be small. The plane we went on to Antwerp only had nine passenger seats. It felt surreal. It was such a dinky little plane, with two propellers on each wing, and it was very noisy. I didn't think the plane was going to make it off of the ground! And I didn't know there was an airport in Antwerp until we got to it.

The funeral was on Wednesday. There was a short service outside, in a cemetery. It was raining and someone had brought along a small dog, which barked incessantly throughout the service.

My Granny, who was really upset and crying, was standing by the guy who was doing the service.

Dad pushed me, in my wheelchair, up to in front of a plateau, which had a black urn on it, and said:

"Dit au-revoir a grand-pere," (say goodbye to Grandpa).

Me (taken aback): "Au-revoir..."

Without saying anything else, or showing any emotion, Dad pulled me back to let other people go up to the urn. Clare and Yvonne went up to the urn together, followed by some other people (whom I didn't know).

Then the guy conducting the service, picked up the urn and pressed something on the top of it (like a cafetiere plunger) and the ashes came out of the bottom of the urn and landed on the grass beneath it.

After the funeral a few people came back to Granny and Grandpa's apartment and had some food.

I felt really sorry for Granny who was extremely upset and kept crying. Never had I seen her like this. She was normally a strong, no nonsense type of person. I did my best to comfort her.

The next day Clare and I flew home and on Friday I went to school as normal.

I felt a bit upset about Grandpa but I didn't remember seeing my grandparents much (at all) since my parents split up, in the early eighties.

Whenever I think about my Grandpa's funeral I always think of 'Word Up' by Cameo! It was in the charts at the time.

My dad is not a religious person – nor someone who believes in the supernatural world.

The next time Clare and I saw Dad, I remember him saying that on the morning Grandpa died, he (my dad) woke up suddenly and sat up in bed as he heard Grandpa calling out to him. Bear in mind, Dad lived in Liege and my grandparents lived in Antwerp.

I feel my book has just entered The Twilight Zone!

It was at about this time that Clare had a new school friend called Hillary. Hillary didn't get on well with her adopted parents, whom she lived with, so she often stayed with us. Hillary was at our house so much of the time that she became like part of the family. She was a nice girl.

It is difficult to describe how my relationship with Mum deteriorated because it happened gradually over so many years. However, it started to go downhill when I was eleven or twelve. Mum knew I wasn't very happy. She said it was because I wasn't trying hard enough in life (because I didn't have any friends at home).

She was of the opinion that I should join a chess club. I had joined a lunchtime chess club at middle school but I didn't find it interested me.

The truth is, I had friends at school but I didn't want to bring them home because of what happened with Nathan.

Martin did come over to my house once and I went to his house on one occasion. Likewise, with Ricky, I went to his birthday party, where I met his sister, Claire. And I remember going into Shoreham with Ricky one weekend.

When I was in my early teens, I started to have different hairstyles. First, I had a crew cut, then a flat-top and then gelled spiky hair.

Mum was still saying I wasn't trying hard enough in life – and often said her life was harder than mine – because she had to look after me and Clare, and that she had a lot to worry about because we didn't have much money. In my mind, I didn't understand how she could compare her life to mine.

Mum was always very critical about my appearance. It was her little comments which got to me, over so many years. At the time, her comments just washed over me:

"You haven't tucked yourself in properly at the back."

"You can't dress yourself properly."

"You haven't combed your hair properly."

"You can't go out looking like that."

Mum didn't like my nervous cough. She used to compare me to Grandad (bearing in mind that my Grandad had a loud chesty cough, he wasn't a very nice person and nobody really liked him).

Her way of dealing with my nervous cough was shouting at me, "Don't cough like that – Grandad."

I sometimes replied back:

Me: "It doesn't help you shouting at me."

Mum: "It makes me feel better."

Whenever I replied back to her comments, it ended up in a shouting match. Hence, I often didn't say anything in return.

There's no doubt that my relationship with Mum didn't feel very pleasant at the time. However writing about it today – and having learnt so much about people and human behaviour in the last four years – I understand Mum's concerns. I dearly love my mum and I know she has always wanted me to be as able-bodied as possible.

One of the things I have learnt about (and to do) since getting into property investment is – living in the present moment – which has really helped me.

People worry about things which, either have happened in the past or things which they think are going to happen in the future. But here's the thing: the past cannot be changed and the future hasn't happened yet. The only time which matters is right at this very moment (as you are reading this right now).

When you live in the present moment (which takes knowhow and practice) you became at peace and there is NOTHING to worry about.

Shortly after I turned thirteen years old, Mum, Clare and I went to see the film *Top Gun*. I was a bit nervous that I wouldn't be allowed in to watch the movie because it had a 15 certificate. To my surprise, nobody questioned how old I was.

It wasn't until a few days later, when I thought about it, I began to think and realise that I could get away with some things – due to my CP. I knew some members of the public were apprehensive of me and found me intimidating.

In December 1986, Clare and I went to see A-ha at the Brighton Centre. It was really good and the first concert we went to.

Over the next fifteen years or so I went to see various pop artists in concert – at the Brighton Centre or Wembley – including; Prince, Madonna, INXS, Paul Simon, Bryan Adams, Aswad, Roxette and Suede.

Sometime in 1986, Mum started a relationship with Dean, who had been her evening class Communications teacher. (They obviously communicated very well together!) It was nice to see Mum happy. At first she was acting like a lovesick teenager, which was a bit irritating, but after a while she calmed down and it wasn't annoying anymore. Clare and I got on alright with Dean and in early 1987 he moved in with us.

One Saturday morning in February 1987, I asked Hillary if she could help me to go into Shoreham (in my wheelchair) and buy a Valentine's present for a girl at school. On the way into Shoreham, Hillary kept asking me, "Who's this girl at school then?"

"Just someone I know..." I kept replying.

We went into Woolworths and I bought a red rose. When we came out of the shop I said to Hillary, "Here you are, I bought this for you!" and I handed Hillary the rose.

I didn't know how she was going to react but I think she was a bit surprised because all she said was, "Oh, thank you, that's very nice of you." I felt disappointed that nothing else was said about it. Hillary knew me well enough to know what I was like – and I liked her.

By now, I could walk up to fifty yards or so – but there was an issue with the way I was walking. I wasn't putting the heels of my feet on the ground. I was walking on my toes with my heels up in the air. I went to see a surgeon in Brighton a few times. The surgeon recommended that I had an operation to release/lengthen my Achilles tendons. He could perform the surgery at Chailey Heritage (a school and hospital in East Sussex for disabled children).

I had the operation on 6th March 1987. I remember the date because it was the day that Townsend Thoresen's Herald of Free Enterprise capsized in Zeebrugge (the boat crossing we used to do when we lived in Belgium).

I recollect waking up after my operation and seeing the news on the little TV, next to my hospital bed. A few days before my operation, Dad mentioned he might come over to England to see me. Had he had done, he might have been on the Herald of Free Enterprise.

I would have liked Dad to come to see me after my operation but didn't think he was going to, so I wasn't too disappointed when he didn't.

While I was in plaster I was unable to walk or to put much weight on my feet. Hence, I had to use my lightweight wheelchair. The plaster went up to just below my knees. It was a pain being in my wheelchair the whole time. For one thing, it made my hamstrings really tighten up. I didn't like the confinement, the restricted movement in my legs and not being able to walk. But I knew it was only going to be for a few weeks.

Clare and I went to stay with Dad while I was in plaster, during the spring half term. It was weird, I think Dad carried me up the stairs (and/or Clare did).

Granny was staying with Dad and Yvonne at the time, too. She wasn't her normal self anymore since Grandpa died. Granny had become incontinent and, to make matters worse, she had had some sort of injection in her right arm, which had gone wrong somehow. This resulted in her arm being constantly puffed up and virtually unusable.

We were all sitting at the kitchen table at Dad's one evening, eating dinner, when, for no apparent reason, Granny wet herself. It was a very upsetting situation. Here was the lady who used to make the loveliest waffles. She could no longer look after herself and went to live in an old people's home shortly after.

Up until the age of fourteen, I used to get upset when Clare and I said goodbye to Mum at Gatwick, on our way to stay with Dad. I think it was because Dad was a lot more strict than Mum (and because I didn't get on that well with Yvonne). However, by the end of our stay with Dad (a week or two) I often wanted to stay a bit longer!

I will never forget when Clare and I were on our way home to England, after staying with Dad one time. We were sitting on the plane about to leave Maastricht Airport, when one of passengers had checked in their luggage but hadn't turned up on the flight.

Therefore, everyone had to get off the plane and go and identify their luggage, which had been put outside.

I started to panic because I wanted to get off the plane but couldn't move or go anywhere because my feet were in plaster and I was unable to walk. I felt trapped. Clare had to go and identify our suitcases but I didn't want her to leave me on the plane – so I burst out crying.

The reason, I thought, the missing passenger hadn't got onto the plane was because they had put a bomb in their suitcase – and I was going to be the only person left on the plane – with the bomb!

I had the plaster taken of my feet in June, using an electric circular saw. The heat and vibration I endured having the plaster removed this time, was as frightening as when I came into contact with a circular saw years earlier, after the first operation on my legs.

After having an operation on your feet or legs, you need a few weeks of intensive physio to learn to walk again. I stayed at Chailey Heritage for a few weeks, where I had daily physio.

By mid-July or August, I was back at home and had made a full recovery.

This was the time when I went into Worthing, by bus on my own, to see the latest *Jaws* film at the cinema. Liz was staying with us at the time, who was a little concerned about me going into Worthing by myself. I knew I could do so. I thought of it as a little adventure and challenge. I knew I could make it over the footbridge, and to the bus stop in Shoreham High Street. I knew people would help me get my wheelchair on and off the bus. And I knew the bus stopped on Worthing seafront opposite the cinema. It was easy. Liz was going to pick me up after the film.

Sitting in the cinema watching the film, I felt a sense of achievement but I also felt sadness. I was unhappy because I had no friends to go to the cinema with. I thought: *When I'm older I'll have a girlfriend, then a wife and I'll be happy.*

I was now walking with my heels flat on the ground, following the operation on my Achilles tendons. However surgery of that nature wasn't 100% guaranteed (every action has a reaction).

Although I was walking with my left heel flat on the ground, I was walking on the inside of my left foot – and dragging it on the ground, with every step.

This led to me having to wear orthopaedic Adimed boots, and a small calliper on my left leg, for the next nine years. The shoes looked like white trainers. They had Velcro and were easy for me to put on. The calliper was made of one strip of metal, which plugged into the outside of my left shoe, and it went up to just below my knee, where there was a Velcro strap. My left shoe also had a small buckle strap which did up around the lower end of the calliper.

The calliper wasn't uncomfortable and it was fairly unintrusive, as my trousers went over it. Obviously, it was visible when I wore shorts in the summer – but I didn't mind.

The calliper helped to straighten up my foot but I still dragged the inside of it a bit when I walked. I remember wearing the calliper with black shoes as well over the years.

In September, a new girl called Sabrina started at school. She wore bright red lipstick and was a year older than me – and I thought she was SO hot! Sabrina said a few times that she wanted to play with my fishing rod. I didn't realise what she meant at first! She never did.

At home, when I got to thirteen or fourteen-years-old I started mentioning, "I would like a girlfriend..." and "When I find a girlfriend..."

I remember Mum replying once, "You'll never get a girlfriend looking like that."

The hurricane of October 1987 blew in the conservatory at the front of our house. It was a bit freaky and scary, as it woke us up in the middle of the night.

The next day we went for a short drive. It was like something out of a science-fiction film; houses had been partially destroyed, overturned cars and caravans, uprooted trees and bottle-banks in the middle of the road.

Builder Barry lived in the road behind ours. He boarded up our conservatory and rebuilt it a few weeks later, once the insurance claim had been approved.

This was about the time when Grandad went into hospital with a chest infection. We drove up to London on three consecutive Sundays to see him and to be with Nan. It was virtually impossible to have a conversation with Grandad because he was so deaf and his health was deteriorating week by week. When we got home from seeing him on the third Sunday, Nan phoned and said that Grandad had died shortly after we had left the hospital. He was eighty-nine years old.

The following week was an unusual one. On Tuesday, I was booked into Brighton Hospital for an operation to unblock my nose as I was unable to breathe through one of my nostrils.

As I lay on the bed, about to be wheeled into the operating theatre, I said to Mum, "I'm scared..."

Mum replied, "Just think about what I've been through the last few days." It was then that 'Turn Back The Clock' by Johnny Hates Jazz came to mind, as it was in the charts.

I was meant to come out of hospital on the Thursday, but that morning, I wasn't being cautious enough walking around the ward and I tripped on a telephone lead and fell over, which caused my nose to bleed. They, therefore, made me stay in hospital another night. My carelessness annoyed me.

On the Saturday Mum, Clare and I drove up to London for Grandad's funeral. I didn't go to the funeral because my nose surgeon advised me to take it easy and not to get stressed. Hence, I stayed at Nan and Grandad's with my great aunt Doris.

I had always felt sorry for my Nan because she was a lovely person and hadn't had an easy life with Grandad. She had had a rough upbringing too; her mum died when she was two-years-old, she inherited a wicked stepmother, got caned at school for being left-handed and lived a poor life in the East End of London. Now Nan could go out with her friends more and enjoy herself.

In early 1988, Mum was determined to do something about my education. She could see I wasn't going to get anywhere staying at the secondary school I was at. We visited two disabled boarding schools, both of which took several hours to get to. The second boarding school we went to had some very bright kids and seemed far more academic, than the first boarding school we visited, so that's where I was heading to in September 1988.

Out of the two schools, it was an easy decision which one to opt for. Although I wasn't looking forward to going to boarding school – and an all-disabled one – I knew it was the right decision because it would academically push me.

In order for my local education authority to fund me going to boarding school I had to see a school psychologist and a bald guy, from the county council, who reminded me of the headmaster in *Back to the Future*.

It took a bit of time, but once my new education establishment was confirmed things changed a bit at secondary school. No longer was Monroe dragooning me in her office every five minutes. I even took to wearing a light-yellow jumper, instead of my dark yellow school shirts (and tie).

During the Easter holidays I had a week at Hindleap Warren in East Sussex, an outdoor activity centre for disabled kids. The things I did there include abseiling, canoeing and a treasure hunt one evening in the dark. It was fun and Martin was there too.

However, most of the other kids there were far more disabled than I was. It made me feel uncomfortable because I don't think of myself as being disabled – and it made me feel as if I was.

I've always fought against being put in a 'disabled' box.

One of the volunteers that week at Hindleap was Dan, who became a friend of mine.

Also In 1988, Dad got promotion to be the director for an IMS subsidiary near Paris so he moved to France (with Yvonne and Juliet).

Two days before Clare and I went to stay with him in France, Dad phoned us and said that Granny had died. It was a bit unexpected.

On the way back from picking up Clare and I at Charles de Gaulle airport, Dad told us that early the next morning he was going to Belgium to attend Granny's funeral and he would be back in the evening – he said Clare and I were to stay with Yvonne. Hearing Dad say this really frustrated me because he didn't ask us if we wanted to go to Granny's funeral. I felt like

Clare and I weren't given the choice. Instead it felt like Dad just said, this is what's happening...

I would have liked to have gone to Granny's funeral. I was also sad to have lost three of our grandparents in quite a short space of time, and while Clare and I were still relatively young.

Dad had moved into a rented house on the outskirts of Paris. The house was in a neighbourhood where it was an offence for people to mow their gardens on Sundays! Dad said he worked hard during the week so wanted a bit of peace and quiet at the weekends.

Back at home, at fourteen, I became very interested in cars (knowing I could start learning to drive at sixteenyears- old), and Mum let me change gears for her when she was driving. It got to the point where she didn't need to tell me when to change gears or which gear to go into. I knew when to look at her foot on the clutch. Mum said it was like driving an automatic car!

Sometime in 1988, Mum and Dean split up. I felt guilty because I thought part of the reason why they separated was due to Dean finding it hard to cope with me.

Clare came with me to see *Oliver Twist*, the end of year play at my secondary school, where James played the lead role.

I didn't want to leave my friends, nor was I looking forward to going to boarding school, but I knew, educationally, I would do better there.

During the summer Dan took me, and another lad with CP, on a week's canoeing holiday in Plymouth. At the time, Dan lived in Kent and Mum dropped me off at his house the day before we went Plymouth. To avoid traffic Dan wanted to leave the next morning at 4.00 am! So that's what we did – in Dan's puke-coloured Morris Marina – and we arrived in Plymouth at 8.30 am. The canoeing place wasn't open yet so we had some breakfast and went to the cinema. We had a great week.

I'm still friends with Dan today. He lives in Hailsham, which he once described as 'the armpit of Sussex'!

That summer, hoping to do some work experience at Southern Sound radio, I wrote to Chris Copsey (who was the programme controller of the station, as well as being presenter of the breakfast show).

A few days later I phoned the Southern Sound office number and asked to speak to Chris, to chase up the letter I sent to him. I felt VERY nervous phoning the radio station because I thought I had to really impress the people there – I felt the fear and phoned them anyway.

I called them several times. On each occasion, they said Chris had my letter and was going to call me back. It was disappointing that I never heard from him but I felt really good that I had the courage to phone the station a number of times.

Before starting boarding school in September, I had my braces taken off my teeth and wore a retainer at night for a while thereafter. It was really nice not having tramlines and elastic bands in my mouth anymore. My mouth had been a bit congested!

Soon after writing this chapter, in early summer 2013, I posted the photo of Martin and me on Facebook. It prompted an online conversation between Emily and I about our school friends who had Muscular Dystrophy. I then said that I was writing a book about my life and, as Emily is into literature, asked her if she would like to read my book. She's read the first three chapters and given me good feedback.

Not having seen Emily since I left secondary School in 1988 (apart from bumping into each other at a Manic Street Preachers concert), I asked her if she could remember what I was like when I was in my early teens. This is what she came back with:

'At school I remember both your walking and your speech being hard work (at least they looked that way to me). And yet you didn't compromise, you didn't use a wheelchair unless you had to. I think perhaps this sometimes inconvenienced others, who would rather have hurried you along in a chair. I remember you climbing the steps onto the school bus every day, because why shouldn't you if you could! You were willing to take your time, and make others wait! I remember how people struggled to understand your speech but how you persisted with making yourself understood; a lesser person might have withdrawn and not bothered speaking much.

And the things you do now – you aren't following a typical course. You're not just trying to be a disabled person who gets by, content with coming up to the mark of what an average person does. You're striving to go beyond that; to do things that most able-bodied people will only dream of (property investment, writing a book etc). You're not content to take a typical disabled path, or a typical abled path. You want to follow 'The Patrick Path'. For me, that's the kind of uniqueness I see in you.'

Chapter 5

On the afternoon of Sunday, 25th September, 1988, Mum drove me to my new school. Needless to say, I wasn't looking forward to being at boarding school. On the several- hour drive we were listening to the Radio 1 Top 40 Chart Show. When Bruno Brookes played the melancholic 'He Ain't Heavy He's My Brother' by The Hollies it made me burst into tears.

(The song had been reissued after its use in a TV advert for Miller Lite. The reason it made me cry was because I preferred Budweiser!)

Me: (crying) "Please don't make me go to boarding school. I don't want to go."

Mum: "I knew this was going to happen. It's the best thing for you. You weren't going to get anywhere at your old school, it really is for the best. And you can come home at the weekends."

My new school was on two sites – the lower school (for school years one to four) and the upper school (fifth and sixth form).

As I was starting in the fourth year (the year you started your GCSEs), Mum and I arrived at the lower school. The lower school had a few 'houses'. I was in Fleming House, which comprised of two boys' wings and two girls' wings. The boys were downstairs, which was good because we didn't have the hassle of using the lift.

In my first year there, I was on a wing that comprised of three bedrooms, which had adjoining doors and a bathroom off of the two end bedrooms. There were three boys per room. To start with, I was in the middle bedroom, which included a fat kid who snored so loudly that it kept me awake at night.

The staff in Fleming House were nice people. My wing leader was Susan and there was also another lady who worked on the wing, called Brenda. Fleming's housemaster was a guy called

Henry, who was a top bloke because he treated everyone like adults.

I found the layout of the lower school bizarre. Fleming House was at the other end of school to the dining room, where we ate all of our meals. To get to the dining room we had to go outside, along a brick-laid walkway, which had a ceiling but no external walls. The school classrooms were situated along the walkway, on the way to the dining room. It was often cold getting around the school in winter time and the classrooms weren't very warm either.

To make matters worse, the dining room was down a long steep slope. It was so steep that I didn't have the coordination to push myself (in my lightweight wheelchair) up the slope. It mystifies me why nobody suggested I use a scooter or an electric wheelchair. It would have made my life a lot easier.

I don't think anyone has ever appreciated how difficult it was (and is) to push myself in my wheelchair.

Each meal started, and ended, with a member of staff saying grace. People just used it as a signal to start eating and to leave the dining room.

The food was actually quite good. At breakfast there were cereals, porridge and a cooked breakfast. We had a choice of two or three meals at lunch and dinner time.

All of the tables were round and seated six people. There were five of us at our table and we always sat at the same table with the same people. Often a member of staff from Fleming House or a teacher would come and sit with us.

At breakfast and dinner there was a pot of tea on each table. Being a coffee drinker, it annoyed me. I always went to get coffee sachets and a flask of hot water from one of the side tables.

All the plates, bowls, cups and mugs were plastic. Every so often the kitchen staff would clean everything with bleach. It wasn't uncommon for my mug of coffee to come with an aroma of bleach!

It took me many months to settle down and get used to life at boarding school. I was never really happy there. To say I didn't like it is an understatement.

In hindsight, I wish I had had a different mindset to boarding school and allowed myself to enjoy it more.

To begin with, I was immensely homesick which made me emotionally very weak and vulnerable.

I was in class 4a, which was the top class. The kids in my class were extremely bright, which made them very competitive. It was the type of class where people wanted to be the first person to shout out the answer to a maths question. As far as I can remember there were ten of us in the class.

It took a few weeks but the first time I was the first person to shout out the answer in Maths, I stunned and silenced the class. It felt so good! And it earned me some respect among my classmates.

For the first time in my life, I was being pushed academically – and I was being pushed so incredibly hard, I didn't know what had hit me. However, I knew I was intelligent and wasn't going to let my classmates deter me. I felt I HAD to compete with them.

Our form tutor in 4a was Alex Livingstone, who was a top, top, bloke. He was far more relaxed than all of the other teachers and treated everyone like adults. Alex also helped me a great deal.

There were four form groups in my year – 4a, 4b, 4c and 4o. Some of the kids in 4o were the type of people who can't be bothered to work in life and learn something.

Between 4.30 and 5.30 pm every day was prep, an hour's homework in your form group. Some of my classmates and I often did more than an hour's homework. I had so much work to do.

One thing I wasn't expecting to happen at my disabled boarding school was to be bullied. I had fifteen-year-old boys with haemophilia punching me in my arms and legs, people with MD, in their electric wheelchairs, ramming into me (in my wheelchair) and spitting at me (because they didn't have the strength to do anything else). I even had a dwarf punching me.

It felt surreal and so alien to me. At secondary school I was always helping people and they looked up to me. Here, I was a homesick wimp. I didn't understand it at first. I had to toughen up and stand up to my bullies.

Interestingly, nobody in my form group bullied me. All the bullies were in the lower classes of the fourth year.

It is horrible thinking about the bullying culture at boarding school. A lot of the kids had been there since primary school age – and a fair few of them didn't come from a loving family. Therefore, it is kind of survival of the fittest.

I hadn't come across people with haemophilia before and they appeared to be able-bodied. Haemophilia (A) is a disorder which impairs the body's ability to control blood clotting, due to a factor VIII deficiency. In other words, when a haemophiliac at school (aka haemo) started to bleed, they needed to have an injection to stop bleeding – and they went around in a wheelchair, with one arm in a sling, for a couple of days.

Disclaimer alert! I'm not a doctor and am not very good when it comes to injections, blood and guts.

I don't remember how or why, but within a week or two after starting at boarding school I moved into one of the end bedrooms in Fleming House. It was a lot better because I was getting to sleep easier and I got on well with my two new roommates – Gareth and William – who were both in form 4b. Gareth and I became good friends and he helped me to overcome the bullies. He mainly used a wheelchair and could walk a bit.

A good thing that I found in Fleming House was the level entry shower in the bathroom. The shower was easy to get into and it had a seat to sit on. All there was at home was a bath, which was difficult for me to get into and kneel or sit in.

The school day was made of forty minute periods, with five minutes of 'travelling time' between each one. However, most lessons were double periods – one hour and twenty- five minutes. This made the lessons very long.

I was doing five GCSEs: English, Maths, Science, Computer studies and French. I really struggled with English and Maths – especially Maths.

To start with, I had English with the rest of 4a – and some of my classmates were also doing English literature GCSE (as well as English language).

The English teacher was a tall lady with knee-high boots. As I don't remember her name, I'll call her Mrs Tall.

I was horrified when Mrs Tall gave me a Thomas Hardy book to read. I had absolutely no interest in reading such a book – and when on earth was I going to have time to read it? It also quickly became obvious that the level of English Mrs Tall was teaching the class was beyond my comprehension.

Therefore, I went into the English class with kids from 4b and it was at the right level of English for me. There were only seven people in the class (two people were slightly disruptive). The teacher was a guy who wore a leather jacket and who liked going outside for a cigarette during the class. For some reason he didn't last very long. He was replaced by a lady, whose name I don't remember either. As she was shorter than Mrs Tall, I'll call her Mrs Shorter.

Earlier in the book I mentioned that I've only read a handful of books in life and that I would reveal how I've built a wide vocabulary. I also stated at twelve-years-old I started listening to people more intently and that I've learnt a lot from doing so.

The way I've increased my vocabulary is simple and easy. I have done so simply by listening to people.

Recently I learnt the word *vernacular*. Chris Farrell used it in one of his internet marketing training videos. When I heard Chris use the word, I understood what it meant (in the context he used it in) and I thought it was a great word – and I feel like using it now!

I enjoyed Computer Studies; our teacher used, and taught us, a lot of computing vernacular (lingo). I've always liked using computers and anything to do with binary! Mr Lennon was a good teacher, although a bit formal in his approach. He had a bee in his bonnet about people saying things like "it's faster" or "it's better" without any clarification. He would reply "Faster than what... a speeding train?"

I overheard Mrs Tall talking to Mrs Shorter. Tall said, "Listen to this, it's a really good essay..." The essay had been written by Ian (one of classmates in 4a) and included the word *hence*. I understood what *hence* meant so I started using it in my essays! Thanks Ian!

In English, we had to write five hundred word essays and I used an Archimedes computer to do so. At the time I thought five hundred was an awful lot of words. Writing this book, on some days I'm producing a thousand words.

I was always putting new words I was hearing into my essays. However, my spelling was rubbish and I didn't know how to spell some of them. Mrs Shorter was a good teacher but she advised me, "Don't use words you can't spell," which I didn't agree with. I thought, *that's what my spell-checker (on my computer) is for* – so I just carried on using words that I found difficult to spell. Practise makes *perfekt*, right?!!

After a couple of French classes with my classmates in 4a, it was obvious that I didn't need any French lessons. The teacher, Mr Cheshire, advised me to do my GCSE French exams in the summer term (a year early) and he predicted I would get a grade A.

Not having any French classes allowed Alex Livingstone to give me some one-to-one extra Maths tuition. I felt like I didn't know any Maths – not having done any Algebra and Trigonometry, to mention two things. I don't remember what else I didn't know in maths at the time!

Alex Livingstone also saw that I was finding life at boarding school very tough. He told me that I had joined the highest class in the whole of the lower school and the people in it were extremely competitive. I remember Alex saying, "Hang on in there, it will get better."

One day after having my Maths tuition, I went back into my classroom, when my classmates tried to trip me up with French.

A classmate: "How do you say one egg in French?"

Me: "Un oeuf" (which is pronounced differently to oeufs).

Classmate: "What about two eggs?"

Me: "Deux oeufs."

I wasn't going to fall for that old chestnut!

For Science we were split into smaller classes and it wasn't my favourite subject – mostly due to the teacher Mr Beales – who often seemed to pick on me.

I don't know why the lunch break was so long. Lunch was at 12.25 pm and classes in the afternoon started at 1.50 pm – the same time that the Australian soap *Neighbours* finished on TV. Depending on who was on duty in Fleming House, we would normally get to watch the whole of *Neighbours*. This often made me a few minutes late getting to my first class in the afternoon. (I've always fancied Kylie Minogue!)

We had science on Wednesday afternoons and Friday mornings. Arriving a few minutes late one Wednesday afternoon, in front of the class Mr Beales asked me:

"What time do you call this – boy? Are you one hundred and sixty-eight hours early for next week's lesson?" To which I didn't say anything.

I should have replied, "If I were one hundred and sixty- eight hours early for next week's lesson, I wouldn't be late today, would I?"

I've never been a fan of school assembly every morning. In my first year at boarding school I had a choice; I could either go to assembly or have some physio every morning. Obviously, I went for the latter.

I don't remember much about my physio, other than she was good. My hamstrings have always been very tight (hence why I walk with my knees bent). Every morning I used to stand in a standing frame for ten minutes and then my physio gave my hamstrings a further stretch herself.

While I was at the lower school my physio put my legs in plaster of Paris for two weeks, to see if it made my hamstrings any looser – it didn't but it was worth a try. Thankfully, she didn't have an electric saw so she cut the plaster off using a special pair of scissors.

Another thing I found difficult at boarding school was spending most of the day in my wheelchair, it caused my hamstrings to tighten up. Also, being around disabled people the whole time made me feel disabled.

The only time I could really walk was in the evenings. With the school being so spread out I had to use my wheelchair during the day. I often left my wheelchair outside the classroom and walked into it – just to get out of my wheelchair.

The 6.45 am fire drills weren't much fun either!

I obviously already had some good people-skills at fourteen-years-old, I got on well with all of the staff in Fleming House and often asked one of them to push me to and from the dining room.

The thing that I resented the most at boarding school was Saturday morning school. For most kids in life, the weekend starts on Friday afternoon. Not for us. We had to do a twohour activity on Saturday mornings. It wasn't even a proper lesson and I didn't see the point of it.

Rather than being able to go home on Friday afternoon at 5.30 pm, we had to stay until 11.30 am on Saturday morning. I saw it as 18 hours of my weekend being taken away from me. I thought it was most unfair. Mum came to pick me up, and by the time we got home, it was 2.15 pm.

Nevertheless, we could pick, from a small selection, which activity to do each term. The first one I chose to do was model car making because it was run by Alex Livingstone. As a Christmas present that year Alex bought a Porsche 911! Two other activities I recall doing were car maintenance (on a real car) and using a camcorder.

To begin with, I was going home every weekend. After a few weeks my homesickness wasn't improving so Mum decided that I should stay at school for three weeks. I don't think Mum understood how difficult I was finding boarding school because her attitude was that I still wasn't trying hard enough in life. It made me think, *Mum has no idea what I have to contend with.*

My relationship with Mum continued to get increasingly more volatile. Writing about it now, I find it funny that I wanted to go home at weekends, rather than staying at school, considering Mum and I argued at lot of the time. I was emotionally weak and I felt more comfortable with what I knew and being at home.

The problem was; my relationship with Mum was making me ever emotionally weaker. This spiralling pattern went on for many years longer. I didn't understand or realise what was happening at the time.

Over the first two years at boarding school, on average I probably went home every other weekend.

Roughly half the people at school didn't go home at the weekends. On Saturday afternoon the school minibus took people into the town centre – which basically comprised of one longish street. I went into town on Saturdays, mainly to have a couple of hours away from school. Normally, after buying a few bits and pieces, I went to have a coffee and cake in one of the cafés.

My roommates, Gareth and William, went home most weekends. However, when I woke up on Sunday morning, the first weekend I stayed at school, William was putting on his school uniform. I thought to myself, *what the hell is he putting on his uniform for?*

Me: "Morning mate, what you putting on your uniform for?"

William: "For church..."

Me: (my mind started racing) "What do you mean?"

William: "For church, we have to go to church."

Me: "CHURCH...what church?"

William: "School assembly, mate."

Me: "I've never heard anything so ridiculous. I'm not going."

William: (slightly bemused) "You have to, mate. Everyone has to go."

Me: "I don't believe this..."

I got out of bed and went to see the member of staff on duty. I said I didn't believe in going to church and protested a bit. However, I had no choice. I had to put my school uniform on and go to 'church'. I was not happy.

In hindsight, I wish I had refused to go (as a matter of principle most of all). What could they have done to me?

As I said earlier in the book, I have always respected people's beliefs. One of the things I believe is; religion shouldn't be forced upon people – it's a personal choice. I found boarding school far too strict.

My least favourite lesson of the week was the typing class, first thing on Monday morning. They tried to get me to learn to type using more than just my left index finger. It was in a cold, dark classroom, with three girls, and it reminded me of my RE lessons at secondary school because it involved typing something out of a book.

The teacher was a bit of an old dragon and we didn't get on too well. I think my complete lack of enthusiasm and motivation for the class was obvious. I did type using two or three fingers on both hands in that class, but I was slow and it was boring.

I've always been a bit of an old dog when it comes to typing. There's no doubt in my mind that I could teach myself to type using more fingers – if I had the desire to do so. It would help me in the long run. However learning to use speech-recognition software would be better for me. A greater idea is to outsource my typing, by employing a PA.

After Christmas in 1988 and for New Year, Clare and I went to Morocco, on our first Club Med holiday with Dad and Yvonne (Juliet spent New Year with her father). Club Med is a chain of four or five star resorts, where the food is inclusive but you buy drinks using little plastic coloured beads (which you purchase in a bag from reception). It's a good marketing ploy because drinks don't seem expensive when you buy them using plastic beads – especially after you've had a few!

It was a good week's break (of sorts). Whenever I go on holiday I become far more relaxed, meeting and talking to people, while I'm wandering about in my wheelchair. I became buddies with a French guy called Jose, who was working at the resort.

I had really bad asthma on that holiday. It was the first time I had been to a really hot country, where the heat caused me to have severe asthma. I didn't take my inhaler on holiday with me because I hardly ever used it at home. Telling Dad about the problem I was having breathing was really frustrating because he didn't take me seriously. Instead he said, "You're alright, stop being a big baby."

Clare and I shared a room on that holiday. On one night, my asthma was so bad I thought I was going to die. Clare understood how severe my asthma was and was bit worried too. I remember Clare helping me to sit in front of the bathroom sink, where I turned the hot tap on full blast and Clare put a towel over my head so that I could inhale as much steam in as possible. Clare then phoned Dad to come over, who then took my asthma seriously. Fortunately, the bathroom steam worked and I was okay.

The next day, Clare, Dad and I went to see the onsite doctor, who gave me an inhaler. However, the doctor didn't give me much confidence because she was the same lady who we saw smoking around the resort every evening!

The complex also had a nightly discothèque. It was something else which frustrated me about Dad because he let Clare go to the disco – but not me. He said, "When you're Clare's age, you can go to the disco." It made me feel that Dad was holding me back from doing something I wanted to do.

Back at boarding school, I wasn't the only one in 4a to take a GCSE exam a year early. Ian did computer studies and someone else took German. As time went on I became better friends with my classmates.

Towards the end of the summer term in 1989, all of the fourth year went to Churchtown Farm in Cornwall. It was sort of like a science fieldtrip – where I checked how much rainfall there had been one day.

The only other thing I remember about Churchtown Farm was kissing and cuddling a girl a few times, who was a member of staff from one of the other houses at school. All I can recall about her was she had light-coloured hair and wore a yellow jumper. I was fifteen and she must have been in her late teens. The little bit of intimacy I had with her was so nice. Obviously, there was a bit of chemistry during the science fieldtrip!

At the time, I had my GCSE French exams to do so I didn't go to Churchtown Farm with the rest of the fourth year. Instead, a couple of days later Brenda, from Fleming House drove me to Cornwall after I had finished my exams.

The GCSE French exam was in four parts – oral, listening, reading and writing. The speaking and listening parts were a doddle but the reading and writing sections were a bit more difficult especially the written exam because, for some reason, I was handwriting the answers. The exam entailed me and Mr Cheshire sitting at a table in a classroom on our own. Mr Cheshire was invigilating my exam and he was also transcribing my answers, as I was handwriting them, onto another copy of the exam paper. It was a ridiculous way for me to do an exam.

At the time I thought, *it would be a lot easier if I could write my answers on a computer.* Writing about it now, I don't know why I didn't just ask Mr Cheshire for a computer. I think I was in a hurry to finish the exam and go to Cornwall.

I enjoyed the drive to Cornwall with Brenda – and she let me change gears for her! Brenda drove back to school the next morning, and took a naughty kid back with her.

Brenda and I always got on well. I felt a bit sorry for her because she was a single parent with two small children and she didn't have much money.

Back at school, on the last night of the summer term – and because we weren't going to be roommates anymore – Gareth and I decided to stay awake the whole night and talk. Feeling a little tired the next day, I was the one operating the lighting in the school play (using an old BBC computer – very high tech!). I got through it without making any mistakes.

At the start of this chapter, I mentioned that the boarding school was on two sites and the upper school was for the fifth and sixth formers. However, not all fifth formers lived at the upper school. Some people, who didn't have any health issues, lived at the lower school and travelled to the upper school, which took about ten minutes on the school bus. We were known as travellers!

For example, all of the fifth formers who had MD lived at the upper school because they were more prone to getting a chest infection when they got a cold.

In September 1989, Gareth moved to Harrison House at the upper school and I moved onto the other boys' wing in Fleming House.

The school holidays were longer than at normal schools. At boarding school we had eight weeks off in the summer, three weeks at Christmas and Easter (and three half-terms).

Away from school, at fifteen-years-old, I bought *The Highway Code*, quickly read it from cover to cover and memorised the minimum stopping distances. I was so eager to start learning to drive that I had an hour's lesson on Goodwood Racetrack (no, not in a Formula 1 car! In a normal car), near Chichester.

I came away from the lesson thinking that the driving instructor was an idiot! He wasn't sure if I would be able to learn to drive a car and said he thought there was only a fifty- fifty chance that I would do so. It didn't deter me because I *knew* I could learn to drive. He just made me even more determined.

In 1989, Liz, John and Becky moved back to the UK, as John's job on the travel magazine in Hong Kong ended. As we were living in their house and all a close family, Liz, John and Becky moved in with us. The house was big enough and it was good. Mum, Liz and John had always got on extremely well together. Damian and Keith were still working in Hong Kong and returned to England about a year later.

At some point around that time, Mum bought an Amstrad PCW 8256 word processor (one of those cheap, greenscreened, all in one jobbies). It was good value for what it was. I used it during the school holidays and found the keys on the keyboard were light and plasticy.

During the Easter holidays, Liz and Mum went on holiday together somewhere – so John allowed Clare and Becky (both seventeen), to have a party in the house! I was going to be in charge of playing the music for the party, using the Akai stack system and powerful speakers which Dad bought me for my fourteenth birthday. *The stereo is still in perfect working order, would anyone like to buy it from me?*

We invited about thirty people. Clare and Becky also invited all of our neighbours (which is always a good idea when you're having a party because they can't then complain about the loud music – but one of them still did!).

On the evening of the party, John, always a bit of a lark, went upstairs to bed before the party even started. More people than we invited turned up, which got a little out of control but not too much. Everyone seemed to be getting off with somebody – apart from me. Which hurt me a bit but I thought to myself, *I'll have a girlfriend and wife when I'm older...*

The upshot of the party was Clare got her first serious boyfriend (Paul), Becky ended up with a bloke too – and the vegetable seeds which John had planted in the back garden, for the summer, got stampeded on, trashed and beer infested (by beer cans which had been thrown onto the vegetable garden)!

Clare and Becky had some clearing up and explaining to John to do. I just played the music!

Once again, over the summer, I wrote to Chris Copsey, asking if I could do some work experience at Southern Sound. Exactly the same thing happened as the previous year. I built up the courage and phoned the radio station a few times, they said that Chris would phone me back but he never did. It felt even more disappointing than the last time.

Mum thought I should do something else so she helped me to get three weeks' work experience at the local district council. I worked in the Environmental Health Department, which gave me a flavour of wearing a shirt and tie every day and working nine to five – although I did 9.45 am to 4.30 pm. Someone from home dropped me off and picked me up every day. I got paid £50 a week.

Most of the work I did at the council was mundane; I did something on a laptop database and some manual filing. However, my boss was good. We went out and investigated hazardous incidents that people had reported.

Some nutcase claimed that, "The sea off of Southwick beach has got acid in it. I dried myself off after I went swimming in it and it has ruined my towel."

Why would anyone go in the water off Southwick beach? It's a shipping lane for container vessels to get in and out of Shoreham Port!

I will always remember the summer of 1989 for two reasons: 1) I spent it smoking cigarettes! 2) Sue and Jane Meadows came to stay with us one weekend.

Every lunchtime, while working at the council, I went in my wheelchair and sat outside the nearby café, having a sandwich and a cigarette or two.

When I first started smoking, I didn't hold cigarettes correctly and I burnt my middle finger on the end of the cigarette! It soon taught me to hold them between my index and middle fingers.

It was John who started me off smoking; when I went somewhere in the car with him, earlier that summer. I was moaning about Mum being horrible to me. I think he felt a bit sorry for me because his response was, "Here, have a fag," and he gave me one of his cigarettes! I started going out in the car with John more often after that!

I went into several newsagents to buy cigarettes that summer – nobody questioned my age.

Mum and I weren't arguing all of the time at that point. We had the same sense of humour and did get on about half of the time.

The reason why Sue and Jane came one weekend was because Mary, our American neighbour when we lived in Belgium, also came to visit us. (Mary now lived back in the USA.)

We all went for a walk along Brighton beach, where there are plenty of souvenir outlets. It was a sunny day and Mum was pushing me in my wheelchair. I was moaning about the sun being in my eyes. Unbeknown to me, Jane snuck off and bought me a pair of sunglasses!

Jane was such a sweetheart. I was fifteen and she was sixteen (and was secretly smoking at the time too!). I regret not telling Jane, then, that I had always liked her – and not staying in touch with her. Some years later, Mum heard from Sue that Jane had got married and had children.

In August I received my French GCSE result by post. Everybody was expecting me to get an A. What did I get? Grade B.

At first, I thought it was a misprint and that a mistake had been made (denial).

I managed to speak to Mr Cheshire on the phone, during the summer. He said it was my reading and writing which had let me down a bit. I was disgusted with myself and thought, *if I can't even get an A in French, what hope have I got in life?* I felt I was a complete failure and thought I was going to be a laughing stock back at school, because I knew the other two people in my class, who had taken a GCSE a year early would have gotten a grade A (anger).

Then, I let it go and my grade B didn't bother me anymore (acceptance).

In 1989, Clare passed her driving test, Dad bought her a two-year-old Peugeot 205, and she started college in Hove.

I think Hillary went to the same college. However, at some point, Clare and Hillary stopped being friends. I don't know why their friendship ended because I was at boarding school at the time. It made me feel a bit sad because Hillary was a nice girl and I always felt a bit sorry for her, being adopted.

I wasn't looking forward to returning to boarding school in late September 1989 but at least I was feeling more comfortable about it. I knew what to expect and my homesickness had dissipated.

I was on the other boys' wing in Fleming House now and sharing a room with Harvey, who was in one of the lower classes than me in the fifth form. He didn't appear slow or stupid and we got on alright as roommates.

The wing leader was a nice lady called Eileen. There were six of us on that wing (two of whom were my classmates) who were travellers, going to the upper school every day. Straight after breakfast every morning, we got onto the school bus and went to the upper school. We returned to the lower school, after prep, at about 6 pm.

The upper school was much easier to get around because the dining room, and all of the classrooms were in the same one building – and it wasn't so spread out as the lower school. As travellers, we had lunch in a small annex off of the main dining room. I became friends with Aled (a technician at the upper school) who usually had lunch with us at our table.

I was in form 5a with all the same people, and had the same classes, as the previous year. However, I somehow escaped the dreaded typing class!

I have known a fair number of people with MD and remember some more than others (especially my friends from secondary school). Another person who had MD was Danny Tompsett, who was in my tutor group. Physically, Danny was much stronger than other boys with the same condition and age as him. I particularly felt sorry for Danny because he was so desperate to find a cure for MD. It makes me feel lucky having CP.

One afternoon a week we had games/PE and, in the fifth year, I did weightlifting. At fifteen-years-old I could benchpress ninety-five kilos. The bloke who 'taught' weightlifting wasn't my favourite teacher in the world.

Travellers were seconded to one of the upper school houses during the day, where we could go at break times, for drinks and biscuits, and after lunch. At first, I was seconded to Harrison House, where Gareth lived. However, Harrison wasn't my favourite house, partly due to it being down a steep slope. I wanted to be part of Drake House – so I asked to be seconded to it – and I was. Not before the housemaster of Harrison House kindly pumped up my tires to help me on my way!

Drake was a much nicer and more grown up house. The kids in it tended to be older and had a lot more freedom than in the other upper school houses. Also, the people who lived there had their meals in Drake House too (being a traveller, I still had to have my lunch in the main school annex). Drake House was newly built and it had satellite TV. I stayed over in Drake House one weekend, it was good.

My abiding memory of Drake House is going into it, through the electric sliding doors, and seeing 'Nothing Compares 2 U' by Sinead O'Connor on MTV. The television was at the front of Drake House and virtually every time I entered the house, MTV was on and they were playing 'Nothing Compares 2 U'. MTV had that video on such high rotation. It is a great song (and video).

Something I wasn't expecting was another shocking and deeply personal event to occur in my life. When I first thought about writing this book, I was hesitant to include what I'm about to disclose to you – but I got over it years ago and it doesn't bother me anymore.

The incident took place sometime during the autumn term in 1989. I'm not sure whether I was fifteen or sixteen. However, I think I had recently turned sixteen (because I don't remember being fifteen, at the time).

It happened in Fleming House one evening when I was sitting in my room, on my bed, listening to the radio. A boy called Freddie entered my room and said he was looking for Harvey (who wasn't in the room). Freddie was in Harvey's class and he lived in another house. I had never spoken to him before. Freddie then started asking me very personal and suggestive questions – and, before I knew what was happening, Freddie molested me. And then he left my room.

It was something which happened really quickly and felt very surreal. He was only in my room for two or three minutes.

I went into complete shock and all of my body felt numb for several days. I felt like my body, and to some extent, my mind had been violated. I find it difficult to describe how it happened because it took place so quickly and unexpectedly. During the molestation, I remember thinking, *this is not happening... how can this be happening to me?*

It must have happened on a Friday or Saturday evening because the next afternoon, dazed, I was sitting in Fleming's communal lounge with the TV on, when Freddie came over to me. We had this small exchange of words, before he left:

Me: "I feel awful."

Freddie: "How do you think I feel?"

I think he was coming to see if I was going to report what had happened. Obviously, I thought about doing so. But the problem I had was that I felt guilty and partly responsible, because I didn't stop it. I also thought it would be my word against his.

Therefore, I didn't tell anybody about it. Instead, I kept it bottled up inside me for years. In hindsight, not reporting it turned into a HUGE mistake of mine, later in life.

Over the next few weeks and months I felt a range of emotions; guilt, shame, confusion. My confidence plummeted and I became even more of an insular person. I ended up linking the incident to my friendship with Nathan. I still didn't understand why my friendship with Nathan had occurred, nor did I know why Freddie had come into my room – but in my mind, both events were of a gay-ish nature. This led me to become sexually confused over the next year – until I had rationalised what had happened with Freddie. (I don't recommend sexual confusion; it's not a pleasant state to be in.)

The event with Freddie cast a shadow over the rest of the academic year for me. A few months after the incident, I had another short exchange of words with Freddie. It took place at the end of one day at the upper school. I was on my way outside to get the bus back to the lower school, when I went past a classroom which Freddie was in, by himself:

Freddie: "Have you got a minute?"

Me: "Fuck off."

Unbeknown to me, right at that moment, Alex Livingstone was walking up behind me and heard what I said:

Alex: (shocked) "What did you say?"

Me: (extremely embarrassed and gasping for air) "I told him to fuck off."

Alex: "Why did you say that?"

Me: "Er, er, I don't know."

It really hurt me because I knew Alex really respected me. In writing this book, it has dawned on me that Alex gave me an opportunity to report what had happened. At the time I was too emotionally weak and didn't have the courage to tell Alex

I don't remember whether it was that academic year or the one after, when Freddie was expelled from school – after a few people reported Freddie for molesting them. Interestingly, they were all severely disabled boys. Although he used a wheelchair, Freddie wasn't as disabled as the people he abused.

I have never thought of myself as being severely disabled – but I know that I am. It is a question of perception. And perception is reality.

After reading this, I think people may wonder if I have ever had any anger towards Freddie. I haven't really. I did feel more comfortable when he was expelled – because he was no longer around school.

I overcame it in 2000, once I understood why it happened. Up until that point, I still felt partly to blame and also thought of it as something unfortunate that happened to me in the past. Shit happens in life, it's how well you deal with it that matters. I now know I didn't deal with it very well.

The mistake I made was keeping it all bottled up inside me for years. It led to what I consider to be my biggest mistake in life. I feel if I had spoken to someone about it sooner my life would have gone along a happier path.

Shortly after my sixteenth birthday I received a letter from the Belgian army, calling me up to do my military service! How on earth they got my address in England is a mystery. Mum sent the letter to Dad to deal with!

During the Christmas school holidays, over the New Year into 1990, Dad, Clare and I went on another Club Med holiday, to Tunisia. For some reason Yvonne didn't come with us. It was a much better holiday than the previous year! I took two inhalers with me and kept my asthma under control.

On that vacation, I met Kirstie, an Australian skier (some Australians do go *skiing in the snow!*). We stayed in touch for a while afterwards. Having just Googled Kirstie, I see she's now an Australian Labor Party politician – I would vote for her!

When we stayed in Tunisia, Dad and I shared a room. Dad still came out with the same line, "When you're Clare's age you can go to the disco too." Which frustrated me even more than it did the previous year because I didn't know why he felt the need to hold me back.

I was now sixteen and could start learning to drive. However, because I was at boarding school and doing my GCSEs, I agreed with Mum not to start having driving lessons until the summer holidays. Still, it didn't stop me from thinking about what car to buy. Dad advised me to get an English- built car because spare parts for it would be cheaper (and it would make the car easier to maintain). Therefore, I planned on getting a second-hand Ford Fiesta.

Back at school, my roommate Harvey went into sickbay with flu for five days. I had built a good rapport with the lady who was on night duty that week; she brought me a mug of coffee in bed every morning, while Harvey was ill. I was a bit dismayed when he came out of sickbay because my morning mugs of coffee in bed ended!

Later that year, I had to pay daily visits to the school nurse for her to rub cream into my buttocks, after my mishap with boiling water! It happened in the dining room one evening when I went to get one of the flasks of hot water for my coffee. So that my hands were free to push my wheelchair, I always held the flask, upright, between my legs/knees. On this occasion I failed to notice that the lid on the flask hadn't been shut properly. Consequently, boiling water poured onto my wheelchair cushion and onto my buttocks. I don't know how the water missed my manhood – it isn't that tiny!

During one half term in 1990, I went to stay with Dad (without Clare). A few days before I left, Dad phoned me to say that he and Yvonne were splitting up and he had bought a house that he was going to be moving into while I was staying with him.

Dad and Yvonne had been together for nine years and it was strange to see how they parted; I helped Dad pack his stuff up, his removal guys were there, and we left Yvonne, at the old house, packing up her things. Dad just said goodbye to her and he showed no emotion. It seemed an amicable separation (mostly on Dad's part).

We drove to Dad's new house with the removal lorry following us. Dad said, to avoid any speed bumps (for the lorry), he wanted to follow a route he wasn't 100% sure of. We went over one speed bump, which annoyed him ever so slightly, to the point where he apologised to the removal guys when we got to the new house. It reminded me of my perfectionism.

Later in this book, remind me to tell you why I have always thought that it's important for me to be a perfectionist.

In the latter end of that academic year, we had to do an individual project in computer studies, which went towards our GCSE grade. I messed up my project by not planning it and making it too complicated. We had a choice of building a system using a spreadsheet or a database. I opted for a spreadsheet system. I knew I hadn't started it off very well but thought I could recover the situation – by making it more complicated! I knew I should have used a database! By that time, I had no time left to start it again. Hence, I felt disappointed with GCSE grade D for computer studies. I didn't do too well in Science either – but my grade D (or even E, I don't remember!) didn't surprise me.

In Maths and English, my teachers put me in some sort of band and I got the highest grades I could achieve in both subjects.

In English I got grade C, which pleased me. It was a real achievement because I had worked extremely hard writing essays over the last two years and my written English had really improved.

Although I got the highest grade I could in Maths, grade D, I felt disappointed because I had worked very hard in Maths too. One of the GCSEs I did the following year was Mature Maths.

I find it funny writing about it now because I've always been good at Maths and computers.

As the school year drew to a close, I asked if I could move to Drake House in September, when I started living at the upper school. Instead of my requested house, I went into Shackleton.

At the start and end of each school holiday I was taken to, and picked up from, boarding school by a taxi firm based in Shoreham. The guy (Frank) who usually picked me up from school was the owner of the company. I had built a good rapport with him over the previous two years, and he told me a bit about his business and how to run a taxi firm. It gave me an idea at the end of my second year at boarding school. Being sixteen years old, I wanted to leave school and go to work for Frank, in his office, organising all of his taxi drivers, telling them all where to go!

The summer of 1990 sticks in my memory for being the time I started learning to drive. My instructor, called Eddie, was very good. I learnt to drive in an automatic Austin Metro. The car was fitted with hand controls. Most people tend to think of hand controls in a car as being very complicated and expensive things but the ones I used (and use today) were simple.

The main hand control was a push/pull lever to the right of the steering wheel, which I used with my right hand to accelerate and to brake. I pulled the lever to accelerate and pushed it to brake. The hand control ran underneath the steering column and had two metal rods. One of the rods was affixed to (the piece of metal which ran down to form) the accelerator pedal. The other rod went to (the metal piece just above) the brake pedal.

The other hand control I used was a stick on the steering wheel, which allowed me to steer the car using my left hand. The stick was detachable and Eddie attached it onto the steering wheel when I drove the car. (If you visualise a clock-face, the stick was at ten o'clock.)

The accelerator pedal was also detachable. Removing the pedal was good for my size 44 shoes. It allowed me more room to rest my right foot and ensured I didn't accidentally hit the accelerator pedal with it.

I had two driving lessons a week over the summer and learnt to drive around Hove. After a few weeks, my driving was progressing well but I came across an issue when practising an emergency stop. I wasn't bad at pushing down on the hand control to brake, but my reflexes in my right hand weren't quite as sharp as they needed to be and I wasn't braking as fast as I needed to.

Therefore, I said to Eddie, "Why don't I try braking with my left foot?" (using the pedal). So I did.

It soon become obvious that I had no issues braking with my left foot – I was (and am) incredibly sharp doing so. Every time I practised doing an emergency stop, thereafter, it made me laugh out loud because I had overcome a potential problem so effectively and easily. (Had I not been able to brake using my foot, I would have simply improved the reflexes in my right hand.)

Shortly after finding the new way of doing an emergency stop, I decided to always use my left foot to brake – and only used my right hand to accelerate. Today, I sometimes brake using my right hand – I still have the option do to so and because I can.

Another thing I did during the summer was phone a load of insurance companies, to get an idea how much car insurance would be for me on a two or three-year-old Ford Fiesta. I phoned so many companies and they all quoted close to, if not over, a thousand pounds. There was no way I could afford that. I had to find a solution.

I was receiving Motability allowance and had heard about their scheme of leasing a car for three years. At first, I didn't think it was a good deal because I would have forfeit my £120 allowance per month. It equated to £4,680 over the three years and I wouldn't own the car at the end of it. However, now that I knew that owning a car would cost me £3,000 in insurance alone, I looked into the Motability scheme. I found out that I wouldn't have to pay any insurance, tax, repairs or servicing – and a brand new Fiesta would only require an initial down payment of a few hundred pounds. I had found the solution!

Summer 1990 was also when Damian and Keith moved back from Hong Kong together with Camille, Damian's Cantonese wife-to-be. There were nine of us living in a five-bed house! We all got on well and it worked.

We carpeted the garage, which became Damian and Camille's room. The area between the kitchen and the garage (where the washing machine and tumble dryer were) had a toilet, that John extended into a shower room.

Keith and I shared a room. When I was at boarding school, Keith slept in the bed, and when I was at home at the weekends, Keith slept on the sofa in the living room! I don't think Keith minded that much, as he was into watching late night TV and videos. I said goodbye to walking up the ladder into my bunk bed. Keith and I were a bit old for it.

Liz and John had been living back in England for over a year now. Both of them were in their early fifties, and Mum was in her forties. The three of them had been looking into and were planning to start a business. They had found a niche for a subscription based newspaper, for people in the UK, who wanted to go and work overseas.

In the lead up to starting the business, Liz and Mum did a 'back to work' evening class. Mum hadn't been out to work since she did a temping job, before Clare and I were born.

The thought of starting a family business really excited Mum. She changed from being slightly negative and lethargic into a very positive and dynamic person. She was really into listening to Zig Ziglar and other positive thinking cassettes tapes. Mum and I were getting on much better.

Sometime after finishing the evening class, guess what Mum did? She started a relationship her evening class teacher! Neil was a bit older than her and he had a slightly warped sense of humour. However, he was harmless and a good-hearted fellow.

I don't recall Neil and Mum being together for that long – a few months maybe. Neil went back to an old girlfriend of his and then regretted it afterwards, when Mum wouldn't get back with him. Nevertheless, they remained friends. Neil turned out to be a manic depressive – he would spend months on a frantic high, 'bouncing off the walls', and then months feeling really down and depressed. I felt sorry for him.

It didn't deflect Mum from her really positive and dynamic streak. She was doing extremely well.

Back at boarding school in late September, once again I was feeling more positive than the previous academic year. Now in the sixth form, I knew it was my last year at boarding school. Also I knew it wouldn't be long before I took my driving test. I was going home virtually every weekend and having a driving lesson.

I was now living at the upper school in Shackleton House. Like in Fleming House, Shackleton has two downstairs boys' wings. As a sixth former, I was expecting to have my own bedroom. However, when I arrived at Shackleton House on the Sunday evening, I found I was on the wing with all fifth formers – and I was sharing a room with a kid who seemed unintelligent and immature – and who was totally dependent on others. I wasn't too pleased. Someone had obviously got my age or my year wrong.

It didn't matter. Within a day or two I was moved onto the other wing and into my own room. My room had a walk-in cupboard, which stored spare bedding. It meant that people sometimes came into my room to get something from the cupboard. However the cupboard was by my bedroom door and it didn't bother me that much.

I found the staff in Shackleton weren't as friendly as in Fleming House. The housemaster was new . He came from working in some sort of borstal and I thought he was far too severe in his ways.

It was disappointing not to be living in Drake House and I thought about asking again if I could be transferred to it. The reason I didn't ask again was because Shackleton House was part of the main school building and was close enough to the dining room for me to walk to it – therefore I didn't use my wheelchair so much as in the two previous years.

On reflection, I should have made another request to go into Drake House. Not least because there were two wheelchair-bound guys (I'll call them Bill and Ben!) on my wing, who were a year older and bigger than me, and I didn't get on so well with them. They both could drive and each had a VW Golf.

As sixth formers, we didn't wear school uniform anymore but we were expected to wear a shirt and tie. I thought it was stupid and unjust because sixth formers at other schools could wear what they liked. Don't tell anyone, but I sometimes got away without wearing a tie!

I don't remember what happened to my classmates from 5a. I know some of them went onto college.

Something which has baffled me, writing this book, is that I can only remember taking two GCSEs in my final year – Mature Maths and Office Studies. I'm thinking that I must have done more than two subjects. But maybe I didn't – because I was doing the two GCSEs over one year.

Academically, my last year at boarding school was by far the easiest. I picked Office Studies because it sounded logical and easy – and it was! We had the subject at least four times a week and two teachers for it – Kevin and Tom – who were far more easy-going and relaxed than other teachers at school. I stayed in touch with Tom after I left boarding school and we went to see the band Roxette at Wembley together. Writing about it now, I don't know why anyone would go and see Roxette in concert – but we did!

For Mature Maths I had the same teacher I had had for Maths in the previous two years. I found he was always a bit too formal but still a good teacher. Mature maths was easier than regular GCSE Maths.

In the autumn term of 1990, my wheelchair started hurting my back because I had outgrown it. A new wheelchair was needed so I got a red and black Swede Elite (it's the same wheelchair which is living in the boot of my car today and currently has a puncture. I'm in no hurry to get it mended but will do so before my next holiday).

The wheelchair has got a holder on each anti-tip bar to put my crutches in. When I first bought it, the wheelchair had two thin pieces of Velcro, on the back of it, to hold each of my sticks in place. The Velcro didn't prove to be a secure method because the Velcro straps would often come undone and my sticks would fall out.

This was often a pain at school when nobody was around to tie my crutches back up. It meant I had to do so myself; by getting out of my wheelchair, walking to the back of it by holding onto it, pick up my sticks and do the Velcro back up, then walking round to the front and getting back into my wheelchair. It took a lot of energy – I didn't have my crutches to lean on!

Something I remember happening often in my last year at boarding school, and less so in the previous year, was someone dying. It was nearly always someone with MD. When someone passed away, each housemaster would gather everyone round and formally tell people. We already knew they had died, even if the person was part of another house. The school wasn't that big and rumours would spread. And of course, the person wasn't at school anymore.

Every time someone passed away I felt grateful that I have CP and it made me think about all of the friends I had with MD at secondary school. I thought they must be dying too. It was a horrible feeling and difficult to describe. Although I never liked boarding school, in a way, I felt pleased to be there, rather than at my previous school. I don't know how I would have coped 'seeing' my friends die.

A person who I saw more often around the upper school than at the lower school was Mrs Collins, the deputy head of the whole place. She regularly spoke to me in the corridors but I got the impression that I wasn't her favourite person! She wasn't my favourite person either! I think Mrs Collins saw me as a nonconformist.

To call me a rebel at boarding school, I think would be untrue (at least not the kind of rebel I had been at secondary school). On the contrary, I was unconfident, a bit of a wimp and tended to keep myself to myself most of the time. In spite of this, I wasn't shy about voicing my opinions on Saturday school, 'church' on Sundays, having to wear a shirt and tie in the sixth form and about the general strictness of the school.

Back at home, one Saturday morning in November 1990, I took delivery of my red, three-door, brand new Ford Fiesta! I thought it was so high-tech (albeit plasticy!) with electric windows, central locking and a button on the dashboard which opened the boot. The car was my pride and joy.

I hadn't taken my driving test yet. Hence, on the first couple of occasions I drove my car as a learner driver Mum accompanied me. It was an absolute nightmare because Mum kept criticising my driving and shouting at me. We ended up screaming at each other on both occasions – and agreed that she wouldn't come out driving with me anymore.

The local Ford garage had collected my car from Cardiff or somewhere and got the hand controls fitted, in Surrey, on their way back. I don't know why I hadn't arranged for the hand control people (Brian Page Controls) to also make me a detachable accelerator pedal. It proved to be a mistake.

As I was slowly pulling into our driveway, after the second drive in my brand new car, my right foot accidently, and slightly, hit the accelerator pedal. Consequently, I scratched the right rear wheel-arch of my car on the brick-built post, leading into our driveway.

Can you imagine how I felt? I burst into tears. I was devastated. I felt like I had messed up and ruined my lovely new car. I 'beat myself up' for days about it and I felt useless.

However, I knew what I had to do. Within days the scratch was fixed and Brian came to Shoreham to make the accelerator pedal removable. I then overcame my mishap by letting go of it.

Brian adapted the pedal by sawing the metal stem (above the rubber bit of the pedal) in half, and then re-attached it using a nut and bolt. It wasn't rocket science, it was metal work! I could then remove the pedal.

Liz offered to become my co-pilot and I drove round Shoreham Beach with her on numerous occasions. I did fine – and there wasn't any shouting involved!

After getting my car in November, I had decided not to go to Club Med with Dad and Clare that year (they went to Mexico). My driving and passing my test were more important to me. Also, I was a little annoyed with Dad for holding me back from doing things on holiday.

Tuesday, 22nd January 1991 was the day I passed my driving test, on my second attempt. Passing my driving test and having my car at school was a real achievement and it made me feel really good.

My first test was in December (in Eddie's car). I didn't make many mistakes in the test. I just went around one bend a bit too fast and when the examiner asked me to pull over, my front tyre went up the curb slightly. I knew I hadn't passed the test before the examiner told me so. He wore a grey suit and was like a robot; he was very stern and didn't say much.

When Eddie got back into the car he said, "You were unlucky. That was the chief examiner and he's got a reputation for being unfriendly."

Before the test, I was worried the examiner would take me down a steep, 40 mph, hill that I didn't like much. He didn't.

Of course I was disappointed but I knew the only problem I had was that my nerves got the better of me. Eddie helped by quickly getting the date of my second test. I knew what I had to do. I went to see my GP Alison Smith, who gave me some Beta-blockers.

On another occasion when I went to see Alison, she remarked, "My, haven't you got big hands..."

Off the top of my head, I replied, "That's what all of the girls say..." Rarely have I heard someone laugh so much as Alison did.

On 22nd January, with the aid of a couple of Beta-blockers, as I was walking out to Eddie's Metro I was feeling really relaxed and confident. I thought: *Nothing is going to stop me. I'm going to pass my driving test today.*

Mum came out to the car to wish me good luck and had a little white stone in her hand. She said, "Here, you can borrow my lucky stone," as she put it in the right pocket of my jeans. She surprised me because I didn't think she had, or believed, in such a thing.

When we arrived at the test centre in Hove Eddie said, "Try not to laugh when you do your emergency stop!"

I had a different examiner this time. He was relaxed and talkative – I even cracked a couple of jokes along the way! He directed me to go down the steep hill that I worried about last time. It didn't faze me at all, and I went up to forty miles per hour (mph) when I got to the bottom of the hill.

When it came to doing the emergency stop, I slammed my left foot on the brake, and quickly put the handbrake on and the car into neutral. It made me smile! I really enjoyed my second driving test and made no mistakes in it. I knew I had passed it before the examiner said so.

Feeling very pleased with myself and confident, after the guy confirmed that I had passed, I asked him, "Is there anything that I need to improve on?"

He replied, "No, you've done really well. I have never seen anyone do such a controlled emergency stop as you have done."

Passing my driving test had been a dream of mine for years – and it was my biggest achievement in life so far.

Eddie was delighted with me, as were all of my family. I passed my test before my three cousins begun to learn to drive.

When I got home after my test, I had a quick coffee before going for a drive in my Fiesta, on my own for the first time. It was a bit daunting. I drove around Shoreham Beach a few times before venturing into Shoreham town centre. I felt like I had hit the jackpot!

January 1991 was also the month when Liz, John and Mum started their business (a three-way partnership) and they published the first edition of their tabloid-size newspaper on 15th January. The first half of the paper had editorial content and articles on working overseas (which John wrote). The second half contained classified job vacancies (which Mum sourced). Mum also was the one who placed ads in the national press, to get subscribers. Liz managed the subscribers and admin.

They launched the newspaper at the right time and it was a success from the word go. The UK was in recession, the Tory government were in a mess after Maggie Thatcher resigned and John Major took over as prime minister, and the first Iraq war started (Operation Desert Storm). People were interested in fleeing the UK and working abroad.

My family started the business working from home; John used the office at the back of the house, Liz used the conservatory and Mum worked in her bedroom! Also Liz and Mum started the business each using an Amstrad PCW 8256! They were all working hard and loving it. Mum built good relationships with the people she was dealing with in the national press.

After I passed my driving test I bought a car phone. It was cheap to buy and to have installed because it came with a free service for disabled people. I could only dial two numbers on the phone – 999 (emergency services) and 132, which was a special operator who could put me through to a normal phone number, free of charge. I needed the car phone in case I broke down. It came in handy.

At the beginning of February, I drove my Ford Fiesta to boarding school for the first time. It was really nerve-racking because I was only used to driving around town, usually at thirty mph, nor had I driven such a long distance before. But, I knew I could, and had to do it. I felt the fear and did it anyway.

I made the journey on a Sunday afternoon/evening, stopping for a few minutes at the halfway point. Can you imagine how I felt when I arrived at my boarding school? I felt an enormous sense of achievement and I thought it had been easy.

For the first few days back at boarding school I kept popping outside, at break times and lunchtime, just to see my car and to check it was still there! I was seventeen and felt very proud of myself and of my car.

I got on better with Bill and Ben. They were interested in me showing them my Fiesta. In the evenings I went for a drive in my car. It's funny because I felt like I was escaping from prison camp!

Although Bill and Ben were both wheelchair-bound (I think they were paralysed), I felt, in a way, that I was more disabled than them because they didn't have any coordination problems in their arms and hands. I didn't know of anyone else at boarding school who could drive.

Passing my driving test made me feel that I had accomplished something nobody else in my position, with my level of disability and at seventeen, had. I have always strived to achieve 'the impossible' in life.

In the latter part of that academic year, I did two weeks of work experience at Lloyds Bank. Having my car at boarding school gave me confidence and a sense of freedom. While on work experience I thought *I should be entitled to have Saturday mornings off school*. I was being treated like an adult by the bank staff and I wasn't 'going to school'.

Consequently, late one afternoon in my first week at Lloyds, I decided to pay Mrs Collins a visit and went 'marching' into her office (unannounced). I was determined not to walk out of her office until she agreed to what I wanted. It took about twenty minutes and Mrs Collins wasn't very happy to have lost that battle! I didn't care about being at boarding school anymore. I was leaving that hell hole in a few weeks!

All I remember about my work experience is driving to the bank every day and being amazed at how much cash they loaded into the ATM on Friday afternoons.

I achieved grade C in both GCSE Mature Maths and Office Studies. It was the highest grade everyone in my Maths class could get. And probably likewise in Office Studies.

Mrs Collins parting gesture was telling me I wouldn't be able to handle going to college because I wasn't organised enough. I think she was still miffed with me for having two Saturdays off. I've always been an organised person – and went on to do extremely well at college and university.

My time at boarding school was done.

Patrick Souiljaert

Chapter 6

I would like to start this chapter with a saying, a phrase that's commonly used in the property investment community:

If you don't love what you're doing, you're probably not going to be very good at it.

For me, this has been true of writing this book. To put it more positively:

When you love what you're doing, you'll do it very successfully.

It is no coincidence that I did poorly at boarding school but extremely well at Chichester College. This is also true about me working in radio (I'll get to that later on).

* * * *

In early summer 1991, Mum and I went to have a look at Northbrook College in Worthing. We weren't too enamoured by it because classes were spread over several buildings – and over both of its campuses (three miles apart). So we went to see Chichester College.

For some strange reason I was thinking of doing a BTEC course in Business Studies (probably because I had liked GCSE Office Studies).

Moira Mason showed us around the Business and Computing Department at Chichester College. The department was contained in one smallish building (C Block) and there were four disabled car parking spaces right outside it.

Everything was good about it; the building was small enough for me to walk round and all of the staff were very friendly. As we were looking round Moira made a suggestion:

Moira: "Why don't you do the BTEC in Computer Studies (instead of Business Studies)? I think you'll do well at it. I'm the tutor for that course and I also teach the Pascal programming class."

Me: "Alright then! It sounds really good."

Moira: "And the course is four days a week. You get Fridays off in the first year."

Me: (Excitedly) "I don't believe it... you've got to be joking?"

Moira: "No, I'm serious! And what we'll do, we'll make sure that all of the classes are here on the ground floor. It'll make it a bit easier for you."

Me: "I don't believe it... thank you ever so much, it's really nice of you."

Moira: "No problem. We would like to have you on the course."

Me: "I can't wait to start. I'm going to love it here."

I couldn't believe my luck – and I had the whole summer holiday ahead of me. I asked Moira what I should read up on over the summer, in readiness to start the course.

The family business was going extremely well. It was publishing the newspaper twice a month, which was being printed in Oxford.

The business was going so well it enabled Mum to buy a house (house prices had dropped slightly due to the recession, which helped). Now that I had left boarding school, with nine of us living in Liz and John's house – and with it also being used to run a full-time business – the house was a little cramped!

We were friends with the family who lived in the four-bed detached house, two doors away from us. Mum had always liked their house, it was up for sale and Mum was in the process of buying it.

I had a motorway driving lesson with Eddie in my car. We went up the M23 (Brighton to London motorway). I drove to the end of the M23 and back – it went well.

Also that summer, I drove to Oxford and back two or three times, collecting thousands of copies of newspapers. It weighed my Fiesta down a bit but it was fine.

Mum, Clare and I moved into our new house in August. It was a nice property. Downstairs, it had a big kitchen and a lounge/dining room, two bedrooms, a bathroom and separate toilet. Upstairs, there were two bedrooms and a bathroom. Mum and Clare had the two upstairs bedrooms and used the bathroom upstairs. I had the back bedroom downstairs, which was a lot bigger than my room in Liz and John's house.

Our house didn't need any work doing to it apart from the downstairs bathroom, which just had an old bath and sink in it. Mum has always had an eye for interior design so she got handyman Eric to knock down the wall between the toilet and the bathroom – and she drew out the layout of the new bathroom, which included a separate shower. Eric built the new bathroom

Being a visual (and dominant) person, the way things (and people) look is most important to my Mum. I too like things to look good, but being more of an analytical person, practicality is more important to me.

The new bathroom looked posh but its wooden floor wasn't very useful for someone walking with crutches. Walking on wet wood with sticks is like ice skating. I wasn't in favour of having a wooden floor in the bathroom but Mum was of the opinion that I could cope with it.

The separate shower cubical was good. Eric built a tiled wooden seat, at the right height for me to sit on and that I could easily stand up from. The shower had sliding doors which were a bit of a pain because they were stiff to open and close and I had to step over the plastic rail they ran along.

I needed to take my sticks into the shower with me, therefore the bottom of them got wet. The difficulty was getting out of the shower. My wet crutches were virtually useless because they were so slippery on the wooden floor. Hence, I got out of the shower by holding onto the sink and lifting each foot over the plastic door rail, which wasn't easy. I then walked very carefully (so as to not slip over – and by leaning on the cupboard door for support) to the bathroom door. Once I got onto the hall carpet I was alright. However, I occasionally fell over in the process.

Clare started university in the Midlands (and moved into halls of residence) when I started at Chichester College. She split up with her boyfriend Paul sometime that year. Clare was always the dominant person in her relationships and she wasn't someone who tolerated being messed around.

I felt excited and confident about starting college. The course I was doing was a two-year BTEC Ordinary National Diploma in Computer Studies. It was all based around computing and a very practical course. The marking system went up; pass, merit, distinction. Eighty per cent of the final grades each year came from doing assignments throughout the year, whilst the other twenty per cent was from the open-book exams in the summer term.

The drive to Chichester College was twenty-five miles. It took me an hour during the rush hour and forty-five minutes off peak. I didn't mind the journey because I really liked driving my car. I was really into listening to Radio 1 and particularly enjoyed Simon Mayo's breakfast show – especially his 'Confessions' and 'On this day in history' features. When I arrived at college before 8.45 am I waited in my car to hear 'On this day in history'!

I've never been a fan of car stickers, but in 1991 I had a Radio 1 sticker in the top middle of my rear window – together with my small car phone aerial on the top left of the window. I thought it looked really cool! Coincidentally, the red part of the Radio 1 logo matched the colour of my car.

At first I couldn't believe how different Chichester College was from boarding school. The contrast between the two couldn't have been greater. It felt like I had escaped from prison camp and was now at a four star resort.

All of the people on my course were really nice. We all helped each other out and there was no competiveness like there had been in 4a and 5a at boarding school.

The teachers were informal and friendly, we called all of them by their first name. We could wear what we liked. The lessons were an hour long and it wasn't uncommon for us to have an hour or two between classes.

Because the subjects we did were all geared around computing, I found them engaging and I wanted to do well. I worked really hard and achieved a distinction in most of my assignments.

Moira Mason was a top lady and turned out to be one of the best teachers I ever had. Pascal programming was my favourite class. Pascal is a high-level language and an easy first language to learn (high-level languages are more straightforward to understand than low-level languages, which are further towards machine code).

Ranjit, the head of the department, was a good bloke. I don't remember what subject we had him for but it involved writing informal and formal reports. This improved my English tremendously.

Maths was really good as well. I grasped Algebra and simultaneous equations far easier than I did at boarding school. A lot of the work we did in Maths was on spreadsheets and it was fun! Richard took us for computer system architecture. This class was all about binary, logic gates and the like. Richard had the tendency to be a bit light-headed which just added to the enjoyment of his lessons!

I really got into using MS DOS and writing little batch files to perform shortcuts. We also went through a word processing revolution at college. At first we used Wordstar 4 and I quickly learnt all of the keyboard shortcut commands I needed to know. Then came Word Perfect 5.1 (and its blank blue screen) and I learnt another set of keyboard shortcuts.

In the second year, Windows and Word for Windows arrived. At first I was reluctant to make the switch to it. I thought, *there's nothing wrong with Word Perfect, it does everything I need it to do.* Windows looked arty farty to me! However, once I started to use Windows and Word I got used to it.

Another thing I liked about Chichester College was that all our classes were on the ground floor of C Block and I could walk around the building. The only time I used my wheelchair was to go to the canteen. It wasn't a problem because my classmate, Mark, helped me. We got the wheelchair from my car (just outside C Block) and put it back in the car afterwards.

It's only in writing this book that I've realised people at college found me inspirational. The staff bent over backwards to help me. My classmates respected me and I got on well with all of them. People treated me like I wasn't disabled. I felt like I was equal to everyone else on the course. It was a nice environment to be in. It wasn't unusual for me to give classmate, Bola, a lift to Bognor Regis, on my way home.

When I started the course, I didn't have a PC at home so the staff lent me one of those old green-screened IBM computers (with a five and a quarter inch floppy drive) until I got my own PC. Thinking about it, I'm pretty sure Moira lent me the computer when I went to look around Chichester College, at the start of the summer.

In the first year of the course, the staff asked me, and fellow classmate, Michael, to represent the Business and Computing Department at a local careers' fair. The thing I remember the most about that day is sitting behind a desk with Michael in a big hall full of other tables and people. We drank an endless flow of coffee throughout the day: after every cup:

Michael: "D'you want another coffee?"

Me: "Go on then...!"

It was a good thing to do because we kept telling everyone what a great place Chichester College was and handing out leaflets. By the end of the day I felt like I was bouncing off the walls!

The overriding thing which made college so good for me was the fact that I fell in love with Rosie – a girl on my course. It happened in the second year at college but I liked her from the start.

Rosie was about my height (short!), had long brown hair and was natural looking. She never wore any earrings or make-up and tended to wear jeans. Rosie was quite a quiet and unassuming girl. She was the most attractive girl I had ever met.

However, Rosie had a boyfriend (Steve) who, I think, was on another course at college because he came into C Block at the end of the day for her (I'm surprised I never asked Rosie what course Steve was on).

At college, I felt happy and confident but, at first, I didn't have much courage to say anything to Rosie (partly due to her going out with Steve). As the first year progressed, I gradually started talking to Rosie; saying hello to her, asking her how she was and making small-talk with her. It hurt me that she had a boyfriend.

On my eighteenth birthday I was supposed to go to college. Instead most of the day was spend sitting on the toilet! It was on a Thursday and as we had Fridays off college that year, my classmates sent me a birthday card in the post.

That weekend, all my family and I went for a meal at the greyhound stadium in Hove. I sat on the left hand side of the rectangular table and we ate our meal while watching the twelve dog races. Staff came round the tables to place people's bets and there were a myriad of television screens so you could see the races going on, from wherever you were sitting. It was good.

At the end of one race I opened my arms with much glee, thinking the dog I had bet on was the winner. I did this with such velocity that I wacked my left arm on the metal pole at the end of the table (which was holding up the ceiling).

My arm was in so much pain that I immediately went into a deep sweat and felt like I was about to faint. I thought I had broken my arm. (With a high pain threshold, rarely do I hurt myself so severely.) However, my arm felt fine after two or three days. To add insult to injury, it was the wrong dog and I hadn't won the race!

Bizarrely, months later at college, and for no apparent reason, the exact same pain came back. My left arm was so painful I could hardly move it. I do not know how I managed to drive to Worthing A&E for an X-ray (sometimes I think I have an extra bit of inner-strength), I could barely walk with my crutches. The hospital said my arm was just bruised. In hindsight, I could have gone to Chichester A&E – I drove past it every day.

At the weekends I usually went out with my cousins to the cinema or for a meal. We regularly went for Dim Sum on Sundays. On Friday or Saturday evenings we typically went to the local pub known as The Duke, which was a haunt for eighteen to thirty-year-olds to hang out. It was the pub where everybody knew my name!

I've always tended to be a lightweight when it comes to alcohol and am very sensible about drinking and driving. I don't like the taste of beer/lager and I need it watered-down with lemonade! I once made a pint of lager shandy last me six hours!

On the nights that I didn't drive to The Duke, I often drank a pint or two of snakebite and black (half lager, half cider, with a blackcurrant top). It was a potent drink I sometimes drank as an eighteen-year-old.

Damian was in a rock band and sometimes played at The Duke. Keith had a friend, who he knew in Hong Kong, called Malcolm. Malc now lived in Croydon and often stayed at Liz and John's house at the weekends. Malc and I become mates.

On Sunday evenings, Mum and I (and Clare when she was home from university) usually went over to Liz and John's for dinner – or they all came over to our house. It was good.

Over the New Year and into 1992, Dad, Clare and I went to Club Med in the Bahamas. On the way there we stayed overnight in Miami. Early the next morning we flew in a little plane over the Bermuda Triangle to Nassau. Needless to say, we didn't disappear.

It was a really good holiday. I met my good buddy, Jake, there, who was the water sports instructor at Club Med. We got on like we were brothers and he took me sailing on Hobie Cats. A Hobie Cat is a type of sail boat with two hulls. Jake's speciality was making the boat go on its side with the hull up in the air. It was good fun!

Having grown up in California, Jake is an experienced surfer and sailor, who now lives in Hawaii. In the subsequent years since we met, I've been to visit Jake in California and twice in Hawaii. I go years without speaking to him and when I phone him up, he says, "Come to Hawaii tomorrow...!"

I haven't seen or spoken to Jake since 2002 (apart from a few Facebook conversations) but he's now married and has a child. They have just completed a six-month sailing trip around the Bahamas.

Dad and I got on better when we went to Club Med in the Bahamas. He didn't stop me from going to the nightclub that year. I remember getting drunk with Jake and him pushing me in my wheelchair straight down the three steps into the nightclub. I fell out of my wheelchair and hurt my ear – but I was laughing too much to care!

It was to be our last Club Med holiday because, in 1992, Dad was made redundant by IMS (after twenty-five years with the company). It led him to move to the Bordeaux region of France, mainly for the warmer weather. Now in his late forties, Dad met a woman at a show-jumping event, called Marie, and he moved into her house.

Dad had a dark green three piece leather sofa set, that he had bought years earlier when he lived in Belgium. For some reason he didn't want to take the sofas with him when he moved to Bordeaux. Therefore, he shipped them over to us and we had them in our living room. They were nice looking but I didn't like them much because they were the type of sofas you sank into. It made getting up off them incredibly difficult for me. It took a lot of effort. Sometimes, Mum or Clare (if they were around) would pull my hand to help me stand up off of the sofa.

During the first half of 1992 I had a car crash. It happened one morning when I was feeling tired on my way to college. I had had a really bad night's sleep and had only slept for three hours. (In hindsight I shouldn't have driven to college that day).

The accident occurred when I got to the penultimate roundabout before college (there are lots of roundabouts in Chichester). I just didn't spot a car coming round the mini roundabout and I didn't give way to it. The car smashed into my car door (which also shattered the window). The guy I had the crash with couldn't have been nicer about it. The only thing that got hurt was my pride.

I was so annoyed with myself because I'd driven twenty four and a half, of the twenty five miles, and relaxed too much when I thought I had completed the journey.

When I arrived at college, after exchanging details with the nice guy, I phoned Mum, who arranged for the local Ford garage to pick up my car from college and she came to pick me up at the end of the day. I felt embarrassed that people at college saw my smashed-up car.

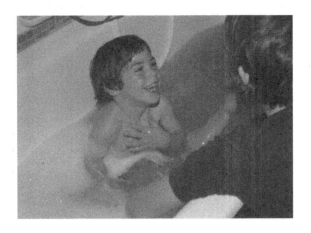

Age 2 or 3

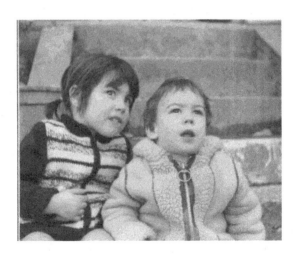

Me and my sister Clare

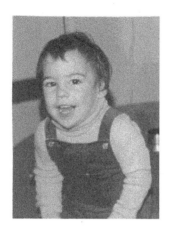

Sitting on the kitchen
table!

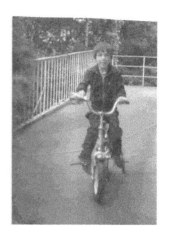

My first
tricycle

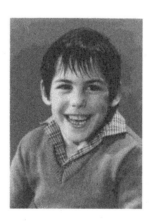

School photo in 1980 (age 6)

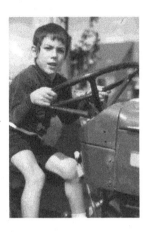

Mowing the lawn

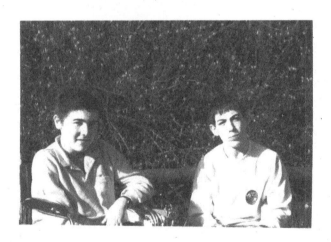

Me and my friend Martin in 1988 (age 14)

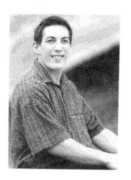

Age 21

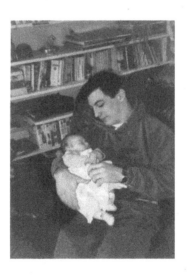

Holding one of my nephews in 1998

Luckily, my accident happened a couple of days before half term, during which time my car was repaired. The accident had shaken me up a bit and I felt nervous driving to Chichester on the first day after half term. But I had no choice – I had to go to college. It was another case of feeling the fear and doing it anyway. It was like falling off a horse and having to get back on it.

The good thing about feeling the fear and doing it anyway is it makes you feel great afterwards.

In 1992 the family business was expanding. They rented an office at Shoreham Airport and took on two full-time, and three part-time, staff. Liz needed a database system to manage the subscribers and Mum required a database to handle her advertisers. Therefore, a local database programmer was hired (called Stuart), who built them a couple of bespoke systems. The business also paid for our summer holiday in Greece that year.

In the summer term at college, having spoken to Rosie a bit I was growing fonder of her. My confidence was good and I feeling optimistic and fairly happy.

When it came to doing the open-book exams towards the end of the academic year, my tutors suggested I did my exams at home! It was an excellent idea. Now having my own PC at home and the house to myself (during the day), I was totally focussed on my exams. I worked tremendously hard and did really well in them.

Throughout her first year at university, Clare hadn't enjoyed her course. Being into horses and having worked at stables, teaching people to ride, Clare decided to do an equine course instead, starting in September.

However, she still had her summer ball to go to and for some reason she invited me to it. Clare now had a new boyfriend, called Rupert. She suggested, so I had someone to talk to, that I invite my mate, Malc. After hiring our tuxedos and all that jazz, I drove up to the Midlands with Malc the day before the ball.

Feeling pretty tired from my long drive, when we arrived at her halls of residence, Clare carried me up the four flights of stairs to her room (my sister is very strong)! That night Malc and

I slept in her room, as Clare and her roommate slept elsewhere with their respective boyfriends.

Early the next evening, after having gone out during the day, Malc and I put our tuxedos on in Clare's room and Clare had her ball gown on. We were all looking good and ready to party! I walked down the four flights of stairs, holding onto the stair rail with my left hand and using my right stick for support. As I reached the ground floor, I looked at Clare a bit oddly.

Clare: "What's wrong?"

Me: "I don't know, my stick feels funny."

As I let go of the handle, the bottom half of my stick fell to the ground whilst the top half of it was still attached to the plastic hoop, which my right arm was in. I had broken one of my metal crutches in half!

It came as a bit of a shock! It was about 6.30 pm and Malc, Clare and I were all dressed up and ready to go to the ball – and I was minus one crutch! We didn't know of any mobility shops in the area and they wouldn't be open at that time anyway. What could we do? Simple – we went to the local hospital, who gave me a new stick. Now, we were ready to have a ball! It was good fun.

Our holiday in Greece that summer had good and bad bits. We all stayed in a self-catering villa. The whole family went apart from Keith for some reason. Damian and Camille were there, Becky had her boyfriend and Clare had Rupert there. I felt a bit left out as usual, but it made me think about Rosie. I had a good feeling about her.

Something really exhilarating that we did in Greece was sitting in a doughnut type of thing in the sea, being pulled along by a speed boat (is it called doughnutting?). Everyone else had a go and of course I wanted to do it (your go lasted until you fell out of the doughnut).

There were two guys operating the ride; the driver of the boat and the other guy at the back of the boat, watching the person in the doughnut. At first the two guys were apprehensive about me having a go and didn't drive the boat very fast. The doughnnut had a handle on both sides of it, and as the ride was quite bumpy, I really needed to hold on with both hands.

However, I kept letting go with left hand, for a second or two, giving them the thumbs up and shouting, "Go faster..." It was great fun, especially once the boat reached full speed, until the doughnut hit a really big bump and I fell out of it. I was hoping for a longer ride but I did well to hold on for as long as I did.

Lying on my back in the sea (with a life jacket on) felt extremely peaceful. Still, I did think, *I hope they're going to come back and get me!*

Another activity which didn't go so well was parasailing. Unlike in Thailand, in 1985, when I took off from the beach with the instructor, in Greece we had to take off by walking to the end of the jetty, which was covered in a sort of green carpet-like material. Rupert had offered to come parasailing with me and, as I wasn't able to walk fast enough, Rupert said he would go behind me, lift me up and he would walk off the jetty.

Can you guess what happened?

As Rupert picked me up (holding me around my stomach) and started to walk forward, he tripped over my feet. We both fell over and the boat dragged us along the jetty and into the sea.

I had cut my thumb while being dragged along the jetty. However, I turned as white as a sheet when I saw Rupert's injury. He had sustained a massive carpet burn all along one of his arms. It was a severe injury, which affected the rest of the holiday. I felt so guilty.

In August 1992, it was really weird the first time Clare and I went to stay with Dad and Marie. It was summer and it was 25 to 30 degrees. Marie was a nice lady and I got on well with her.

Dad had changed and mellowed dramatically. I think working at IMS stressed him out. He had always lived in a modern, light and airy house, with mod cons (the type of property I like). Marie had an old and dark house in a forest area, in the middle of nowhere. The house didn't have things like central heating and a dishwasher that Dad was used to. The kitchen was small and it had a door leading out into the massive garden.

The garden was so big it contained a barn and two horses. Marie already had a horse when Dad moved in and Dad got one shortly afterwards. Marie also had some other animals; two dogs, a few birds, including a peacock that lived outside in the barn.

When Clare and I were there during the summer, the kitchen door was left open a lot of the time and birds just walked in out of the house willy nilly! The living room walls were dark and had three stuffed deer heads on them (not my kind of thing). It was a real old country house.

At the end of the driveway was a long straight road, with trees on either side of it. It wasn't uncommon for a car to hit and kill a deer crossing the road. While sitting in the garden, we heard such an incident occur. Dad and Marie went running down the driveway and came back carrying the dead deer between them. In another part of the garden and away from us, Dad proceeded to de-skin the deer and cut it into pieces, which he then cleaned in the kitchen sink, and put into the freezer. Clare and I were horrified. Even the memory of it is disgusting.

Dad had become country-fied – and swapped his big fat cigars for a pipe. He took to doing the washing-up after every meal. I don't think I had ever seen him do washing-up before.

Marie and Dad's bedroom was downstairs in the house. However, Marie thought it would be better if she and Dad slept upstairs, while Clare and I were there, so I didn't need to negotiate the old staircase. I had no complaints! Marie had three kids (round my age) who we got on alright with.

September arrived and with it the start of the second year at college. It was good seeing all my classmates again. This year, we had some classes together but had to choose one of two streams; COBOL programming or Information Systems.

Initially, I was tempted to pick the COBOL stream; I really enjoyed programming and Moira Mason taught the class. However, I thought COBOL was a bit old-fashioned and I wanted to learn more about databases and spreadsheets – so I opted for Information Systems. At first, I was disappointed not to be in the same stream as Rosie. But it didn't matter.

Later on, during the first term of the second year, Adam, a classmate I got on very well with, said to me, "D'you know Rosie seems like a nice girl…"

To which I replied, "I've always liked Rosie. I've liked her since we started the course last year. I've been wanting to tell her how I feel about her for ages but she's still going out with Steve."

Adam said, "If you feel that strongly about her, you should tell her."

From that moment on, I decided that I was going to tell Rosie how I felt. After thinking about it for a few days, with Christmas coming up, I knew what to do – and I told Adam of my plan.

I was going to write Rosie a letter and make a mix tape of songs for her, that I would give to her on the last day at college before the Christmas holiday.

At the start of December, away from college, a job advert in my local paper caught my attention because it was working at Southern FM (that, until recently, had been known as Southern Sound). The job was 'ad trafficking' (scheduling adverts) and the vacancy listed 'good computer skills' and 'works well under pressure to meet tight deadlines'. I thought, *that's me*! I wrote a letter applying for the job.

Amazingly, I got an interview! It was with Bob Hoad, the managing director. I was a little bit nervous going into the interview but, with nothing to lose, I felt confident. My main selling point was being very good with computers, I would quickly learn the job. I was very enthusiastic and the interview went well. Bob Hoad was a pleasant guy.

I wasn't surprised when I didn't get the job – I was nineteen and had no experience. However, I was disappointed because I knew I would have done a great job as I was very keen to work in radio. On the other hand, I was pleased because I didn't want to leave college and Rosie behind.

I'm proud that my first ever job interview was in radio.

On the last day of college before Christmas, I thought, *I know she's got a boyfriend but I've got to take a chance and tell her how I feel*. In giving Rosie the padded envelope with my letter and the tape I had recorded for her, I said, slightly nervously, "Here's a present for you. Have a happy Christmas." Rosie said thank you, but didn't look that surprised.

I remember on Christmas Day that year thinking about Rosie, feeling a bit nervous and wondering how she would respond to my letter. I thought the best course of action was for me to drink steadily throughout the day. It was going well, until I went to the bathroom, fell against the radiator and burnt my right hand a bit. It didn't bother me – I was drunk!

Because I hadn't had much luck with girls in the past, I decided not to tell Mum or Clare about Rosie (I did mention her to Damian). I had always wanted to find a girlfriend first, before telling Mum and Clare. However, in my drunken state I did mutter something about Rosie so they were aware of her.

Between Christmas and New Year, I received a nice letter from Rosie, thanking me from my letter and cassette tape, and saying we could have a chat back at college. I felt relieved and pleased and full of anticipation.

Going back to college in the New Year and seeing Rosie for the first time was nerve-racking. I said hello and asked her how she was and, as cool as anything, she said, "Let's have a chat." Rosie mentioned that she knew I liked her before I gave her my letter!

Over the next six months, we sat and chatted to each other virtually every day at college. There was a seating area in C Block and we had loads of free periods together. I lost count of the number of hours we spent together and got to know each other. Rosie said she wanted to join the police force at the end of our course.

She was such a lovely girl. We were the same age and had so much in common. Rosie was intelligent, mature and a real people person. My CP didn't faze her or seem to be an issue. I felt so at ease with Rosie. We connected really well.

Over the months, I fell completely in love with Rosie and gave her all sorts of gifts; another mix tape, more letters and sent her flowers. She liked my attention and talking with me.

One day at college I wanted to give Rosie something unique and spontaneous. So I got a few sheets of A4 paper and tore them in half. Then I handwrote a humorous message on each bit of paper, stapled the sequence of messages together and gave it to her.

It was funny because everyone on our course knew that I liked Rosie. The only person who didn't seem to realise was her boyfriend, Steve, who came for her at the end of the day.

In all the months we spent sitting talking to each other, I didn't push things with Rosie. I would have liked it if she had left Steve because she knew that I loved her. However, I didn't want to say something to her that I would later regret.

One day I asked Rosie if we could have a chat in my car – so we did. It was funny because she was at ease but I felt a bit nervous.

Me: "This feels a bit strange."

Rosie: "Why...?"

Me: "I don't know, it just does."

What I really wanted to do was hold her hand and give her a cuddle, but I didn't know how she would react because of Steve. I didn't know what to say to her! So we sat in the car for a few minutes not really saying anything.

Rosie is the only person I've said 'I love you' to. She could tell I was a bit unconfident emotionally. I knew she liked me but she never told me how she felt about me.

I was happy and confident at college and it was no coincidence that two other girls there liked me as well. One of them was Helen, a girl on our course who Rosie used to hang around with. The other person was Caroline, someone with red curly hair, who I saw in the morning when I arrived at college. However, my heart belonged to Rosie.

Caroline would be standing outside the entrance of C Block, having a cigarette. Every day, we made eye contact and smiled at each other when I got out of my car. Then, as I walked into the building we would say hello to each other. I did have a couple of conversations with Caroline, she was from Bognor and her birthday was a day after mine.

Valentine's Day in 1993 was on a Sunday and I didn't feel happy that weekend, as I wanted to be with Rosie. However, it didn't stop me sending her a dozen red roses!

Malc was down from Croydon that weekend and I asked him if he would come to The Duke on Saturday evening with me. He didn't have a girlfriend at the time so he was happy to do so. I went to the pub to get drunk that night. We sat at the bar where I told Malc how I felt about Rosie and that we were so alike, as I downed seven double vodka-oranges in forty-five minutes!

At the end of the night, after most people had left the pub, I went for a wee and decided to crawl around the pub when I came out of the toilet. Malc phoned Clare at home, who came to pick me up – literally! It was the first bit of crawling I had done in years!

The next day made me give up alcohol – and I didn't drink any for seven years. I only really drank alcohol to get drunk. I normally drove everywhere so never used to drink much anyway.

A couple of months later, sitting talking with Rosie at college, she said, "I probably shouldn't say this but we *are* very much alike." It gave me a lot of hope.

While at college I got into politics and current affairs. During the second year, I applied to be in the audience when the BBC's *Question Time* was filmed in Brighton. I went with Damian and it was very interesting. Things really do look bigger on TV! Peter Sissons hosted the programme and Paddy Ashdown was one of the panellists.

Following my job interview at Southern FM, in spring 1993 I joined my local hospital radio station. They had recently moved into the council building where I did work experience when I was fifteen.

I remember going to my first hospital radio meeting. It was on a Thursday evening and there was a lift to the first floor. Not knowing anyone when I arrived I said hello to most of the people there. A few of them looked at me as if to say 'What's a disabled guy doing here?' It made me feel uncomfortable.

The meeting was interesting and informative. The lady hosting it asked for volunteers to help with a street collection they were organising the following Saturday in Worthing. The lady also mentioned that if anyone wanted to be trained on how to use the studio equipment they should speak to Ted, who was standing in the corner at the time.

At the end of the meeting I went over and met Ted. I said hello, introduced myself and asked him if he could teach me how to use the studio. Ted replied, "There's no point in me teaching you how to use the studio because you're never going to be a radio presenter." It brought our conversation to an abrupt end and I let other people speak to him.

As I walked away I thought, *what an ignorant and arrogant arsehole*. However, Ted didn't deter me. I went into the studio, where someone was sitting using the studio desk. Saying hello and building a bit of a rapport with him, asking a few questions, I stood watching what he was doing for a few minutes. *It's easy*, I thought. *I can teach myself how to use the equipment.*

Hatching a cunning plan, I went to see the lady who had hosted the meeting and said I'd be more than happy to help with the fundraising event the following weekend, I then went back to the guy in the studio and asked him when would be a good time for me to come in and teach myself how to use the studio. He said it was normally free during the daytime. He also told me what the keypad code was to get into the studio. *I can come in on Mondays* (my day off from college), I thought.

It was funny at the end of the evening; the main doors out of the building were locked. People were concerned I wouldn't be able to get out of the council! But walking down the fire escape stairs, on the outside of the building (like everyone else), was a piece of cake.

On the Saturday morning, a week later, I drove to Worthing and sat in my wheelchair, outside Marks & Spencer (in Montague Street), raising money. It was good fun and it taught me something. I learnt that people give generously to someone who appears to be severely disabled, in a wheelchair. In about two hours, I filled two collection tins and raised £130.

People were so pleased with how much effort and money had I made, I got a mention during the next hospital radio meeting, the following Thursday evening! Now, I felt comfortable going into the studio and teaching myself how to use the equipment.

It took me two sessions in the studio to learn how to use the equipment. I loved it, so it was easy. There were two CD players and two or three cart (cartridge tape) machines, used to play jingles and adverts.

The second time I went into the studio, an older guy called Tony was there, sorting out the record library. I had brought in a cassette tape to record what I was doing. Tony was obviously watching me and listening. At one point he said, "You've not going to sell that (the tape I was recording), are you?" I thought it was such an odd thing to say.

All I was doing was practising; cueing up one CD whilst the other one was playing, segueing one CD into another, playing a jingle in between songs or over the start of a song, up to the beginning of the vocals.

And that is how I taught myself to use a radio mixing desk (and associated equipment). It must have been around May 1993 because, in the studio, was a CD-single of '(I Can't Help) Falling in Love With You' by UB40.

I didn't last that long at hospital radio because people looked down at me and they didn't like me using the studio.

While I was a college student, I went to the neurological physio department at my local hospital, to have my hamstrings stretched. I was the only person with CP who went there. All of the other patients were old people who had had a stroke.

The stroke patients only needed a few weeks of physio to be rehabilitated. Because I needed my hamstrings stretched on a continual basis, after about six months, the head of the physio department came up with a plan to get rid of me.

She enlisted the help of Remap (a charity of engineers who develop custom-made equipment for disabled people), to make me a device I could use at home to stretch my hamstrings. Along came a guy called Peter, who built me a great big and heavy contraption.

(Peter and I are still friends today. He lives a few minutes away from me and often helps me out with bits and pieces. He's a top bloke).

It consisted of two padded sheets of wood. One about six feet long, (that I laid my back on), and the other two feet long, that connected with one end of the first sheet of wood (in an L shape) that was held together in a metal frame.

I stretched one leg at a time by lying on my back with one leg strapped, using two seat belts, on the upright piece of wood. One strap held my leg against the piece of wood, while the other strap held my knee (and leg) straight. Then a sling went around the ankle of my shoe.

The sling had a rope attached to it which was part of a pulley system. The rope ran through a ratchet above my head, which I pulled and locked in place to stretch my hamstring.

I used to stretch each hamstring for thirty minutes every day while watching TV. It appeared to be a hideous contraption but it provided a very effective stretch.

Either Clare or Mum strapped me into it. Due to an issue with my right thigh muscle which makes my knee turn inwards when tightening up the straps on my right leg, my knee needed to be held down and out with one hand. With my knee turned in, it didn't provide a good hamstring stretch.

Interestingly, Clare did it really well, whilst Mum had a problem with it. It often caused the following type of exchange – leading to an argument:

Me: "Please can you hold my knee out further."

Mum: "I can't do it anymore than I am."

Me: "You can do it more, you're just not trying hard enough."

Ironically, the frustration this caused me made my whole body to go stiff – and caused my hamstring to tighten up!

More often than not, Mum (and I) preferred Clare to strap me in. it seemed to me that strapping me in herself clearly pained Mum.

I used the contraption for three to four years.

Towards the end of the academic year, the Business and Computing Department announced they were launching a BTEC HND course in Business Information Technology in September. It seemed like a good course and a very logical thing for me to do. Therefore, that's what I was planning to do come September.

In spring 1993, a guy I gave a lift to in my Fiesta (I don't remember who) spotted an issue I didn't realise I had. When it came to parking my car, I was finding it difficult turning the steering wheel. The guy suggested that I would find a car with power steering much easier. I contacted Motability, explained the problem and they allowed me to terminate the three-year contract on my Fiesta a few months early.

Shortly before I handed back my Fiesta, the exhaust went on it. It sounded like a race car and I thought it was really cool! Still, I had to get it fixed because it was so loud.

In June I received a blue, five-door, Vauxhall Astra hatchback. I opted for an Astra as its boot was big enough for me to put my wheelchair in, without having to take the wheels off. It came with an RDS radio (which was a new feature to me) and, having back doors, was easier for passengers. Indeed, it was much easier to drive and to park with power steering. I liked it!

Having worked hard at college, I completed my BTEC OND course by achieving a distinction or merit (mostly distinctions) in every module. I felt really happy and pleased with myself.

To celebrate the end of the course, on the last day of college, all of my classmates and I went ten-pin bowling in Worthing. I was no stranger to that bowling alley. The way I bowled was by walking up to the line at the start of alley, then getting down on my knees, and with the ball in the centre of the line, pushing it with my left hand.

Rosie must have seen me bowling on my knees that day.

At the end of the game Rosie and I were talking, sitting opposite each other, when she suddenly gave me a kiss. It felt *so* nice. We agreed to stay in touch and to see each other.

Can you imagine how I felt? I felt like I was in heaven. I couldn't believe that I had managed to 'pull' Rosie (I will describe what I mean by the word 'pull', shortly). Rosie gave me the opportunity that I had been longing for since we started college.

We had spent so many hours together (over the past six months/two years), talking and getting to know each other. We were so alike, my CP didn't bother Rosie and I was completely in love with her (although Rosie was going out with Steve at the time).

I thought to myself, *all I have to do now, is carry on being my natural confident self and keep on seeing Rosie, and our relationship will develop naturally.* However, instead of doing that, I made the biggest mistake (and regret) of my life.

Now – before I go on to say what I did and the consequences – I would like to jump forward to the present day, 16th June 2013 (twenty years later).

I started writing this book in April 2013 and the first five chapters were very easy to write. When I started chapter six, I knew I was going to reach this point which has made the chapter difficult and painful to write.

However, I didn't realise how painful it was going to be. It's not because I'm not over Rosie, It's painful because I wrecked the opportunity she gave me to further our friendship.

Back to 1993 – in the couple of days after we had gone bowling, where Rosie had kissed me, and after we had agreed to see each other outside of college, I felt elated and my mind was racing.

I was feeling so many emotions; I was so pleased that Rosie and I were going to stay in touch and carry on seeing each other. I felt so happy and I became a bit delirious. I felt I had found the person who really *understood me*. Now that our course was over I felt I was free to say to Rosie that I wanted a serious relationship with her – but she was still going out with Steve.

Having got to know each other over the last two years, we connected extremely well together because we were so alike. Rosie knew I loved her and I wanted to have a serious relationship with her. She was a caring person, my CP didn't bother her and she could tell I was a bit weak emotionally. I don't think she would have suggested we carry on seeing each other if she didn't envisage starting a serious relationship with me.

Here is where I made the biggest mistake of my life, and it is something I have always regretted. What I did still horrifies me and I have never told anyone about it before.

I wrote to Rosie, said I was really happy that we going to keep seeing each other and I felt completely at ease with her. I also said that I wanted to tell her something very personal and I was going to tell my family about it as well. On a separate sheet of paper I wrote a little piece about being molested at boarding school.

It was a defining moment in my life – and a mistake that still gives me a pain in my chest when I think about it.

On the same day, after posting the letter, I handed the piece I had written about being molested to Mum. I was standing in front of her as she started to read it, when she said, "Is this a joke?" Because I hadn't told them anything about Rosie, I felt I couldn't tell them about the letter I had just sent to her. I felt like I had nobody to talk to. (My family were initially very sympathetic but nothing seemed to change.)

I then realised what I terrible mistake I had made posting that letter to Rosie. The dread I was feeling became worse and worse. I was shocked by what I had done. It was like having a great idea, up until the time you do it, and then you realise what a mistake it was.

Consequently, I changed overnight. I went from being a happy and confident person, to hating myself and thinking I was a worthless piece of shit. The next day, I became so distraught by what I had done that I couldn't function properly. I had never felt so low in my life as I did then.

To make matters worse, I could have rescued the situation when Rosie wrote me a lovely letter back, saying how sorry she was to hear that, telling me it wasn't my fault and I shouldn't let it worry me. However, by that point, I was feeling so worthless – without thinking what I was doing – I tore up Rosie's letter, it made me start to hate myself even more, and this made me feel that I wasn't good enough for Rosie, so I didn't reply to her letter. For years I have felt bad that I have never apologised to Rosie.

The question is, why did I feel the need to tell Rosie something so very personal?

I think when Rosie kissed me and we agreed to see each other outside of college, it blew my mind and the molestation thing, which I had kept bottled up for over three years, came flooding out of me, I was feeling a lot of emotions, I wasn't thinking clearly and I reached out to Rosie. I lost the plot for a few days. I was emotionally weak and immature.

Twenty years later, I am older and wiser.

The primary mistake I made was not telling someone else sooner about being molested. Had I done so, I wouldn't have told Rosie.

A couple of days ago, I phoned Paul Ribbons, who knows a lot about human behaviour and psychology. Paul and I have a close bond and I can talk to him about anything. He says I sent the letter to Rosie to self-sabotage my friendship with her. The reason being, Rosie was still going out with Steve, I had been hurt in the past and I was scared of being hurt again.

I don't agree with all of that.

I wanted to be with Rosie more than anything in the world. Yes, Steve was an issue for me but Rosie knew how I felt about her and I really don't think she would have hurt me. I think she was waiting to see how our friendship developed at college before leaving Steve. Paul is right to say that I was scared.

If I wanted to end my friendship Rosie by self-sabotaging it, why have I been torturing myself about it since 1993?

One thing I know for sure is sending that letter to Rosie broke my heart. I would have done anything for her. To me, that is true love. I was an idiot to ruin the chance Rosie gave me. But I am only human and I made a mistake.

In 2002, I Googled Rosie's address – and in 2003 I plucked up the courage and wrote to her. I said that I had bought my own flat, was working full-time as a computer programmer and working in radio on Saturdays – but I didn't mention anything about my previous letter to her.

Amazingly, Rosie sent me a really friendly reply, hoping I was okay and mentioning that she was now living with her boyfriend Simon – and she put her phone numbers on her letter.

Hence, one evening, I REALLY felt the fear and called her home number anyway. Simon answered the phone! (I don't know why I didn't phone Rosie's mobile.) I had a short chat with Simon and then spoke to Rosie. She was really nice to me. However, the conversation felt very awkward.

I wanted to apologise to her, all these years later, but I didn't have the courage to bring up the subject. Instead, I asked her if she had joined the police (as she had said she wanted to at college). She said she hadn't. Instead, she worked for an animal rescue centre after leaving college. Rosie emailed me some photos of her and of where she was now working.

That's it regarding contact with Rosie.

Here's the difference between 'pulling' and 'pushing' – which I've learnt through getting into property investment. It's so powerful.

When I was at college I was happy and confident – and without even trying – three girls were attracted to me. I was pulling them towards me.

In contacting Rosie again ten years later, out of the blue, I was kind of 'pushing myself against her'. However, Rosie was very nice about it. I have 'pushed myself against' plenty of other girls over the years who haven't been quite so nice about it!

The law of attraction – I'll give you more examples later in the book.

I still regret sending that letter to Rosie, tearing up her positive reply and not responding to it. What still really cuts me up inside is that Rosie gave me the opportunity to further our friendship and I destroyed that opportunity. I have been torturing myself (and I'm not using the term lightly), about it ever since. It's made me unhappy. It's the reason why I have felt like I haven't achieved much in life.

The other reason it still hurts is because I have been though hellish times trying to find a girl to share my life with. I've been through some painful times in life but, having just written the above, the pain I'm now feeling is excruciating. It feels like the inside of my chest has been ripped into pieces.

I hope you don't mind my honesty and bluntness. Something that I don't think people realise about my life is that most women don't find me attractive. I appear to be very physically disabled – and my affected speech makes me sound like I'm mentally disabled. This reduces the number of women who are willing to give me an opportunity (compared to able-bodied guys). Being rejected by someone is the most painful thing in the world to me.

The most basic human emotion is to love, and to be loved – and to share life with someone.

The good thing in writing about it is I have now realised why I have been beating myself up for twenty years – and I can now deal with it.

One of my greatest assets in life is my mindset – I know that I can overcome anything I put my mind to. I'm Patrick Souiljaert.

I've Googled 'life-changing mistakes' and have read some articles. By reliving regret and what might have been, one is missing out on existing opportunities.

It reminds me of *The Power of Now* by Eckhart Tolle. People worry about either the past or the future – or both. It is pointless thinking about the past because it cannot be changed. Likewise, it is pointless worrying about the future because it hasn't happened yet.

The only time that matters is right at this very moment – NOW.

When you understand and practise this – and live in the present moment – life is bliss because there's nothing to worry about.

I've had short periods of living in the moment but it's something I need to practise more.

The other thing I've found is the following seven-step plan on how to overcome serious regrets *(Source: wikihow. com)* – which I'm going to go through here and now:

Step one – Determine what your regret really is. *Do you regret something you did or something you didn't do? Something someone else did or did not do? A circumstance beyond your control? It is important to step back from the feelings of regret and identify exactly what the regret is.*

I have a few!

I regret keeping things bottled up inside me.

I regret writing to Rosie, without thinking first and about something so personal

I regret destroying Rosie's positive response and not replying to it.

I regret destroying the chance Rosie gave me to further our relationship.

I regret hurting Rosie.

I regret hurting myself.

Step two – Ask for forgiveness and make amends. Apologise for any harm you may have caused others, it does not kill to ask for forgiveness so give it a go! Forgive yourself. Forgiving others will make you happier. Be compassionate towards everyone involved, including yourself.

I've no intention of contacting Rosie again so I am going to write her a note here:

Dear Rosie

I am so sorry for telling you something deeply personal about me. I really didn't mean to hurt you. I wasn't thinking clearly and I made a mistake. It was completely my fault. You did nothing wrong,

Thank you for caring about me and giving me an opportunity. You meant a lot to me.

Best wishes,

Patrick

In forgiving myself, I am going to say: "I am a great person and have got a lot to give. I am awesome."

Step three – Accept the circumstances. Avoid blaming others but rather take responsibility for anything that you could have handled better.

What happened was 100% my fault.

(From the age of fourteen when I went to boarding school, I have always accepted responsibility for myself.)

Step four – Deal with toxic relationships. Sometimes other people cause us to do things that leave us with serious regrets. Do you have a toxic relationship that needs to be addressed or severed?

With regard to my family – I did this in early 2011.

Step five – Grieve for your regrets. When we feel regret, we re-live guilt, sadness or anger over and over again. Allowing yourself to experience these feelings fully with the intention of moving forward can help you stop revisiting them.

I have done this enough over the last twenty years.

Step six – Recognise what you have learned or gained. When you find yourself thinking of the regret, turn your thoughts to the things you have learned and the opportunities that are now yours – even if they are not what you would have preferred. There is always

a lesson even in pain and sadness. Look for the lesson and focus on it instead of what might have been.

Do not keep things bottled up inside of me.

Do not tell people things which I will later regret.

Ask people for help and advice.

Rosie saw the good in me and gave me a chance.

Torturing myself about things I've done wrong does not help anything or anybody.

I am at my most attractive when I'm happy and confident.

I am grateful to have known Rosie.

I am not the guy I was in 1993 – I am older and wiser.

I have got a lot of love and affection to give someone.

Step seven – Write out a plan or agreement for yourself that identifies how you could avoid having this sort of regret in the future.

I will speak to someone when something is bothering me

I will not do something important without thinking or speaking to someone about it first.

That's it! That was easy – and I feel better already.

If you would like to do the same exercise and overcome a regret you may have, I recommend you complete the seven steps in big and colourful letters – then print out the form and stick it on your fridge, in the kitchen. In fact, print loads of copies of your completed form and stick one in every room in your house or apartment. You need to take in the things you have written at each step of the exercise. That's why it's a good idea to stick copies of your form where you will see them.

This exercise is Cognitive Behavioural Therapy (CBT). It's about changing your internal voice and negative thoughts, into positive thoughts and emotions.

If you're reading this and thinking *what on earth is he talking about? I haven't got a voice inside my head.* That's your internal voice that I'm taking about!

Like anything in life, at first you might find it difficult, but the more you practise saying and thinking positive things, the easier it will become. Positive thoughts and emotions will come naturally to you.

I have now finished the most difficult chapter of my book. Awesome!

To remain focused on completing something it's good to visualise the end product. This is how billionaires think. I am now visualising my published book.

Bring on the next chapter!

Chapter 7

Life went on after my disastrous letter to Rosie. What astonishes me is the fact that I went from being happy and confident to hating myself and my confidence hitting rock bottom – and none of my family noticed the change in my frame of mind. I must have covered it up well – much to my detriment.

In summer 1993, Rupert, Clare and I drove to Bordeaux in my new car and stayed with Dad for a couple of weeks. I felt like I was in a daze the whole time. I was glad to let Clare and Rupert do all of the driving to Bordeaux. On the way there we stayed in a cheap motel in Paris for a night or two. Clare wanted to visit some attractions with Rupert. I remember going up the Eiffel Tower. Having been up it before, it was no big deal.

I did do some of the driving once we got to Marie and Dad's house. Juliet came to stay with her boyfriend while we were there. We went to the beach a few times, which included a ten minute drive on the two-lane motorway.

Our first trip to the beach was a scary experience. Clare and Rupert came with me in my car and, as I didn't know the way, I was following Juliet and her boyfriend in their car. They drove so fast along the motorway. I thought I HAD TO keep up with them because I didn't know how to get there. I felt petrified – and I didn't like driving on the wrong side of the road! However, the subsequent trips to the beach weren't as bad as that first time.

On the way home to England, Clare wanted to go and see Yvonne so we stayed the night at her new place, near Paris. Yvonne wasn't as well off as when she was with Dad. She was living in a really small flat and it was obvious that she had a lot of resentment. Despite the fact she was now living with an eastern European boyfriend, who was about half her age.

The ferry crossing from Dieppe to Newhaven was a bit choppy and it made me throw up, in plain view. I felt really embarrassed.

Clare had now finished her equine course but was still living in the Midlands with Rupert, as he was working there. However, Clare did move back home with Rupert some months later.

A few weeks prior to starting the new HND course in September, Mum and I went to see a studio flat in Chichester. I was on Income Support so could have got Housing Benefit to rent a property. However, I was in no fit state and couldn't cope with the thought of living on my own. I just said I didn't like the studio flat – and that was the end of that.

It was much to my shock and horror, when I started the HND, to find that Steve (Rosie's boyfriend) was also doing the course. That was the final straw. It felt like a dagger had been shot into my heart. My whole world was completely shattered. I couldn't concentrate on the course. Chichester College wasn't the same anymore and it was too emotionally painful to be there. I lasted for the first six weeks, until halfterm. The excuse I gave for leaving was that I didn't like the business element of the course.

I felt awful and didn't feel like doing anything anymore. Now I had another thing to feel bad about. In leaving the HND course, I felt like I had failed and that I was a quitter (I have never been a quitter in life). I was now coping so badly that I told Mum I needed help. She thought it was due to me being molested at boarding school and she organised some counselling for me in Brighton.

I had counselling once a week for three months. My counsellor (Jim) was a good bloke but, having had other forms of therapy over the years, I don't think counselling is very effective. All it seemed to entail was me talking and Jim listening. Jim did ask the odd probing question, such as, "How does that make you feel?" I did feel more confident during the twelve weeks while having counselling but quickly reverted back to feeling really low afterwards.

Having said that, all I spoke about in my counselling sessions was about having no confidence and a bit about the molestation event at boarding school. I didn't mention Rosie.

Writing about it now, I find it really strange because the thing I was really upset about was the thought that I had destroyed my friendship with Rosie – which caused me to hate myself. I think I was so horrified about the letter I sent to her that I didn't want to admit it. However, self-sabotage, as Paul Ribbons suggested, may have been the case. I don't know. It doesn't make much sense to me.

Whitney Houston's 'I Will Always Love You' didn't help me get over Rosie when it re-entered the charts in December 1993 (it was one of the songs I put on the second mix tape I made for her). Every time it was played on the radio I had to switch to another station or turn off the radio. Hearing that song was too painful for me.

During the three months I was having counselling, Mum and I went to have a look at Brighton University. Its HND Computing course seemed good and the department was contained in one building (Watts), which was bigger than C Block at Chichester College but small enough for me to walk around it.

Unlike Chichester College, the course at Brighton University consisted of lectures and tutorials (lectures gave the theory which you practised in the tutorials). The person who showed us around and told us about the course said there was a lot of note-taking in the lectures. As I would find it difficult to take lots of notes myself, they advised Mum and I to go and see the university welfare officer, Trish.

Trish was a very helpful lady who suggested I apply for a Community Service Volunteer (CSV) to help me at university. She said that a CSV could go into lectures with me and take notes, and assist me with my typing and generally help me around the university (the canteen was in the building opposite Watts – and I needed my wheelchair to get to it). Trish also advised us that I could get a grant to fund my CSV.

Community Service Volunteers is a national charity which helps disabled people with everyday life. This could be assistance at home, in the workplace or at university. Volunteers normally do a placement for six months or a year and they get their accommodation and food paid for, along with some spending money.

The other thing we spoke to Trish about was the possibility of me living on campus. She said it wouldn't be a problem and she could reserve a place for my CSV too. The halls of residence were modern and the block I was going to be in had six bedrooms and a level-entry shower/wet-room bathroom.

Hence, it was set – the following September I would be starting at Brighton University and living on campus, with my CSV. I felt apprehensive about the whole thing. In the meantime, I applied for two grants: a student one for me and one to fund my CSV. I also contacted Community Service Volunteers regarding finding me university helper (scribe) for September.

Mum and I also had a look at Portsmouth University, which was spread over various sites and didn't appear to be that suitable.

Nan was still living in London and coming to stay with us every few weeks. Something that we first started to notice, probably back at the beginning of 1993, was that Nan was becoming a bit forgetful. It was really strange, she would start a sentence but then not remember what she was going to say halfway through it.

Therefore, sometime in 1993, Liz and Mum took Nan to see Alison Smith, who referred her to a specialist. As we suspected and dreaded, the specialist diagnosed Nan as being in the early stages of Alzheimer's. Although it didn't come as a shock it was very distressing. Nan was a lovely person and she hadn't had an easy life. In early 1994, she could no longer look after herself nor live on her own – so she moved in with us. Nan had the spare room downstairs in our house.

It was around the same time that George (who used to take Clare to school) died. I remember walking into Mandy and George's house after the funeral (for the gathering) and hearing 'Georgia on My Mind' by Ray Charles. It was the first time I had heard it and I immediately thought *oh, what a great song.*

I felt sorry for Mandy after George's death and I went to see her a fair few times thereafter. Mandy and George had always been nice people.

Early 1994 was also when Clare moved back home with Rupert. Clare got an enjoyable job at a stables in Brighton, teaching people to ride horses. Rupert worked in Hove.

During my gap year, I arranged to go and have a look round Southern FM. I met Danny Pike, who was a nice guy and who presented the breakfast show. It must have been around February because 'Come in out of the Rain' by Wendy Moten (a top song) was in the charts. I recall Richard Gwynn playing it while I sat in the studio with him, during his mid-morning show.

Another person I met that day at Southern FM was Gary, the station engineer. We chatted for a few minutes and he told me what his job involved. Gary said one of the things he did was the Saturday evening show, between six and midnight, '100 hits in a row' – and he invited me to sit in on the programme.

I found it fascinating. All of the songs were played off CDs, which were stored in a large rack on the back wall of the studio. The jingles and adverts were on blue cart tapes and it was a presenter-less show – Gary didn't do any links (a link is when the presenter says something on the radio). The programme was simultaneously broadcast on Southern FM's sister-station Ocean FM (in Portsmouth). Therefore, Gary played two sets of jingles – one for each station. (It was in the early days of radio networking!)

It inspired me and frustrated me at the same time (more the former than the latter), because I knew it was a show I could learn to do – and I wanted to do it! However, I got the impression that Gary became bored with me when I went in and watched him on the third occasion! What it did do however, is made me even more determined to work in radio.

The family business was still going well and growing. As Damian was a journalist, he was taken on full-time to assist John on the editorial side of the newspaper. However, this caused a problem for Mum. She often came home in the evening and moaned that Damian didn't work very hard.

She said Damian was often on the phone to his friends, organising his band practice sessions and his social life – and that Liz and John were turning a blind eye to it. I advised Mum to speak to Liz and John about it or not let it bother her – she was still enjoying her job and it was due to the business that she could afford to buy our house (and to pay the mortgage).

Mum did not follow my advice. Instead she did nothing about the situation and it kept 'eating away' at her over a period of months and years. She was regularly moaning to me about how 'Damian is so lazy'. The situation frustrated and upset me because Mum didn't do anything about it – and her positive streak began to fade.

During my gap year, I also worked for the business for a month or two. I didn't last very long because I was mainly doing clerical work which didn't stimulate me at all. Feeling so low, I didn't feel like doing much or working in an office anyway. Also, I could see what Mum meant about Damian not pulling his weight. It made me feel uncomfortable being in the office. I sensed that working for/with my family was not a good idea.

They worked in a smallish, first floor, open-plan office. Together with Mum, Liz, John and Damian were two fulltime and two-part staff. Liz, John and Mum were still getting on very well but there was a hint of friction in the office between John and Mum at that stage. John tended to be the dominant one (in the partnership) and wanted to take the lead and make the decisions regarding the business.

On the ground floor of the office was a restaurant/bar and a flying club. I became a familiar face in the bar, and I built a good rapport with the two guys who ran the flying club. They offered me a free lesson in one of their two-seater fixed wing planes. Despite me feeling it was quite an old plane and likely to fall apart at any moment, it was great fun. We headed east to beyond Brighton's Palace Pier and back again. I found flying the plane easy and thought I could go anywhere in the world in it!

I also got invited to a stag do in the bar one Friday evening – which included three strippers. Being twenty years old, I thought it was excellent. During the intermission, while I was minding my own business and sitting with my back to the bar, one of the strippers came up to me and we chatted for a couple of minutes.

Without warning, she then grabbed my right hand and thrust it onto one of her naked breasts and said I was a sweet guy.

Another thing I enjoyed was going to the local car auction with John, Damian and Keith. John bought a couple of old bangers there over the years! I liked going round looking at all of the cars before the auction began and then found the auctions really exciting. Although I had a nearly new car, I was always tempted to bid on cars and buy one! I think I accidently placed a bid on a car once when I had an itch on my nose!

Damian got an old Ford Escort from the auction, which he and I took for a test drive the day after he bought it. We went to Horsham to have lunch with Camille where she was working. On our way home, the oil light came on so Damian bought some oil at a garage. He then opened the bonnet and poured the oil into the brake fluid compartment! It's the sort of lightheaded thing Damian did. He can be a dipstick sometimes!

It turned into a bit of a nightmare. We waited three hours for the recovery service, who couldn't drain the oil out, so we waited more hours for another recovery vehicle to tow us home. We arrived back at eight o'clock in the evening – and it turned out to be an expensive lunch for Damian!

Something which fascinated me once I started driving and going out in my car was how people's perception of me had changed. Earlier in the book, in my explanation of going to the shops in my wheelchair from the age of twelve, I said how a lot of people saw me in my wheelchair, heard my voice, assumed I was mentally disabled and spoke down to me. Well, when people saw me getting in or out of my car and walking with my crutches they didn't treat me like I'm stupid. When people saw I could drive a car, they realised I wasn't stupid.

Today, when people see me getting in or out of my car and walking about they will often come up and ask if they can help me – rather than avoiding me. It's not unusual for fourteen-year-old kids (and above) to ask me if I need some help.

Isn't that fascinating?

Back in 1994, life at home was becoming more stressful – with Clare and Rupert in the house. Some of the friction was caused by a clash of personalities between Mum and Rupert – and them not liking each other. It seemed to me they were both fighting to have control of Clare.

Mum has never been good at containing her emotions. Although she didn't say it to his face, it was plain to see that Mum didn't approve of Rupert. She thought he wasn't good enough for Clare.

I think at first, Rupert did try to gain Mum's approval but she never accepted him being with Clare. Hence, the two dominant people – Mum and Rupert – always had a fiery relationship.

What I found most upsetting was how Clare changed after she met Rupert. She had always been the dominant person in her relationships and she never took any crap. However, for Clare's relationship to work with Rupert, one of them had to become the submissive person in their relationship – and that was Clare. It was painful to see Rupert boss Clare around. At times it felt like Clare was his servant.

From what I have learnt about people and psychology over the last few years (and studies have shown this to be true), when there is conflict between a mother-in-law and son-in-law – and the mother-in-law tries to break apart her daughter's relationship with the husband – it, in fact, has the opposite effect. It pushes the wife closer to the husband.

This was certainly evident with Clare. Whenever Mum (or I) said anything derogatory about Rupert, Clare would leap to his defence – and they stayed together for nearly twenty years.

My view of the situation was that Clare had chosen to be with Rupert – hence I accepted the situation. I don't think Mum ever did.

By the time I started university in September 1994, Clare and Rupert had moved to Coventry, where Rupert got a job. It was a shame they moved because Clare was enjoying her job, teaching horse riding in Brighton. It also proved to be a defining moment for Clare because she was committing herself to stay with Rupert.

Mum has a very charming side to her. As a visual person, she takes pride in her appearance and has always looked about ten years younger than she is.

In the nineties she had a few platonic male friends. There was handyman Eric, who popped by one evening a week for a coffee or glass of wine. Another person who became good friends with Mum was Stuart, who built a couple of database systems for the business.

Stuart often tried to help Mum set things up on her home PC (over the phone) but she was never interested in learning how to do basic stuff on computers. It frustrated me because it seemed she never tried to help herself. Whereas I have always had the opposite mindset (I've always tried to help myself). Instead Mum would rope me into speaking to Stuart to do things on her computer. Consequently, Stuart and I became friends.

The other guy that Mum stayed friends with was Neil (the manic depressive). Neil seemed to be on a permanent low throughout the nineties and Mum tried to help him.

At one point, when Neil's GP visited him at home the doctor noticed Neil had a Stanley knife on his desk (which Neil used for his work). However, the doctor jumped to the wrong conclusion, thinking Neil might self-harm, and sectioned him into a mental hospital for a few weeks.

It prompted Mum into asking me if I would visit Neil in the hospital, as he felt extremely down. The thought of going to a mental institution didn't fill me with joy but I did it anyway. Neil really appreciated it and I felt like I had done a good deed. I was a bit concerned that on hearing my voice the doctors in the hospital would keep me in there!

Never will I forget Mum saying to me, "The problem with Neil is he wants everyone else to help him but he won't help himself."

Meanwhile Nan's short-term memory was getting worse. Her mind had regressed to when she was a child. She thought her dad was still alive and the one thing she always wanted to do was to go and see him. With increasing regularity Nan would say, "I want to go and see my father in Eric Street." (Where she lived in East London when she was a child.)

When she first wanted to go to see her dad we said, "He doesn't live there anymore..." However, this upset her and we quickly learnt to reply, "We can go and him tomorrow." This seemed to keep her contented.

Over a period of four years, Nan would say three or four times a day, "I want to go and see my father in Eric Street." It was distressing to witness but Nan deteriorated so gradually that it wasn't a shock. She also became a very fussy eater. Anyone who has cared for somebody with Alzheimer's will know how difficult it can be.

When Nan first came to live with us, Mum took her into the office and Liz mainly 'looked after' her by keeping her occupied. As they received a lot of post in the office, Liz gave Nan the empty envelops and she would, very carefully, tear off the used stamps. Nan enjoyed it. She also did other menial tasks, like tidying the store room. Nan liked having things to do.

Looking after Nan was a joint effort. Sometimes, Becky or Keith had her. Sometimes, I stayed home with her. Mum was good with Nan but occasionally, with her short fuse, Mum would shout at Nan. This caused me to shout at Mum (not to shout at Nan), which triggered even more tension at home.

Over the summer of 1994, I received three or four profiles from Community Service Volunteers of potential scribes to help me at university. I remember one profile was of an eighteen-year-old guy who listed one of his interests as seventies music. As I was more into eighties music, I ruled him out!

I decided to go for Andrea, an eighteen-year-old girl from Glasgow. I thought as she had chosen to do voluntary work that she would be a nice and caring girl.

My mindset was different to when I started college in 1991. I wasn't happy or confident. I was anxious about starting university and living on campus. Having always been self-sufficient, it felt weird having to have a helper at university. I was worried that the people on my course would see me as an outcast.

Andrea travelled from Glasgow to Shoreham by train. I recall going to meet her at Shoreham Station on the Saturday evening.

Walking onto the station platform, my whole body was shaking so much that I could hardly walk. Anyway I did it, and once we met I felt much more at ease.

Andrea was a bit nervous too, but she seemed like a nice quiet girl. We went home and Mum had cooked a chicken dinner. That evening Andrea and I chatted before moving onto campus the next day.

Andrea seemed excited to be moving onto campus, whereas it petrified me. The ground floor flat we were living in had six bedrooms – we were two guys and four girls. On the day we moved in, I was so out of my comfort zone that I felt really sick. Unbeknown to anyone, I went into the bathroom and threw up in the toilet. It got rid of all of the tension I was feeling.

The first week on campus was Freshers' Week. The people I was living with were nice and they included me in things. We went clubbing a couple of nights that week and out for a meal one evening. We stayed up late every night in our flat. People came over from other blocks on campus and we drank and partied until the early hours.

I felt like I was just going along with the crowd. I was usually the first person to go to bed.

I was living with at least two nice girls – Sarah, who was starting the second year of my course and long, blonde-haired Joanne. I didn't fancy Andrea, as I found her a bit young and immature (and a bit spotty!).

During Freshers' Week all of my flatmates and I went to the university event where people could join clubs – and I became a member of the Labour party! My membership was short-lived, however, because on two occasions thereafter I went along to the local Union Office and all they got me to do was stuffing envelopes. It didn't stimulate me, nor was it my idea of fun so I didn't go again.

Having dropped out of the HND course at Chichester College I had decided that I had to do well at university and I became a really analytical person. Or rather my analytical side became more dominant than the kinesthetic side (my people-person side) of me.

When university started in earnest, the week after Freshers' Week, I found it was nothing like the time I had at college. All of the lecturers were fairly nondescript and not very approachable (apart from my second year tutor, Liz Matthews, who was good). I didn't gel as well with the people on my course as I had done with people on my OND course at college.

At university there were two guys on my course, both in their thirties, who went around together with an air of superiority, as if they were better than everyone else on the course – and they kind of looked down upon me. It caused me to decide that I had to compete with them.

Another thing I didn't like about university was the lecture and tutorial style of teaching. In lectures, I always sat in the front row (with Andrea taking notes). It meant I sat in all my lectures with nothing to do. I felt like a lemon. Sitting in the front row (because it was easier than walking up the steps and sitting further back), I felt segregated from the rest of the people on my course.

Writing about it now – and having been on a lot of property investment courses (and done internet marketing courses, online), where I've taken notes using my laptop, I realise, when I was sitting in my university lectures doing nothing and not taking my own notes, I wasn't absorbing much information. I retain much more information when I type my own notes.

The subjects at university were pretty much the same ones as I did on my OND at college, they were just taken to a more advanced level.

In the first year at university we did Ada programming (like Pascal, it is a high level language). It was my favourite subject because it was the most practical one.

Like at college, university consisted of doing assignments throughout the course and exams towards the end of both years.

After Freshers' Week was over I became focussed on working hard and doing the best I could on my course. My analytical mind was set to getting good grades and I didn't want to stay up partying until two or three o'clock in the morning anymore.

However, my other flatmates did and because I was living with four girls, it attracted a lot of students from other blocks on campus to come and party in our flat.

We were having a party every night for more than two weeks after our courses had begun. I was going to bed at about one o'clock in the morning – and then getting frustrated because I couldn't get to sleep for the next two hours, due to there being so many people and a lot of noise.

This is how *anal*-lytical I became (and I am embarrassed to admit this). The doors in our flat were all fire doors which closed themselves automatically when someone went through them. I was complaining that people were coming in the flat, and in and of out of the lounge – and I couldn't get to sleep at night because I could hear the sound of the doors closing. Hence, Mum bought some sticky rubber foam and she stuck it on the inside of some of the door frames.

I am not like that anymore!

Andrea was having a whale of a time because she was living the life of a student – and had no course work to do.

The strain started to surface during the second week of my course. I had several 9.00 am lectures. Andrea was tired because she was going to bed at about three in the morning and I, too, was tired, as I wasn't getting to sleep until the early hours. The situation wasn't improving.

By the fourth week it was a nightmare. It felt like taking notes for me in lectures was an inconvenience to Andrea because she had no interest in learning about computing.

Trish, the university welfare officer, got involved and was extremely helpful. Andrea said she didn't want to stay and help me. It made me feel incredibly guilty and responsible because I had picked Andrea to be my helper – and she had come all the way from Scotland.

Trish told me that this sort of thing had happened before and I shouldn't let it worry me – and I would find a more suitable helper. However, it didn't stop me feeling responsible and beating myself up about the situation.

For some reason it was agreed that Andrea would stay for another two weeks until half term.

Life in the flat became unbearable for me. Andrea got on well with the other three girls. It felt like they were all against me and that I was the bad guy. After a few days I couldn't cope with it anymore so I moved back home.

Initially, it was only going to be while Andrea was still there. However, once I was home, in my mind, I had moved back home for good. This caused more tension with Mum. I recall, standing in the hall, having the following heated and repetitive exchange with her:

Mum: "You are not moving back home."

Me: "Yes I am."

Mum: "You are not moving back home."

Me: "Yes I am."

Mum: "You are not moving back home."

Me: "Yes I am."

I felt under so much pressure thinking that everything was my fault and blaming myself, I could barely drive to university. Andrea still came to lectures with me until she left at half term. Although we never argued with each other, the situation felt very tense.

When I moved out of the flat, Trish told me that Andrea couldn't remain living on campus until half term unless I paid my rent to live there too. Just to keep the peace and to not make the situation even more stressful, I agreed to pay my rent, even though I wasn't living there.

I felt under so much stress; Mum and I were constantly arguing and I wasn't concentrating on my university work. The only way I knew how to relieve the stress I was feeling was by throwing up, which I started doing in toilet at home in the mornings.

I felt like giving up – but I kept on going – I was determined to get good grades at university.

I remember going back to the flat on the day before half term to get the rest of my stuff from my room. Somebody had taken off the sticky rubber foam from the living room door frame and stuck it onto the outside of my bedroom door, in the form of a big letter P.

Me: (pointing to my bedroom door) "What's this?"

Andrea: "It's a letter P, for your name."

It REALLY hurt me because it was a sign that the people in the flat didn't respect me.

Writing about the whole situation now, I class moving back home, rather than staying living on campus, as my second biggest mistake in my life. I think had I felt the fear and stayed living on campus, I would have matured, emotionally, a lot sooner.

I think it was crazy that I moved back home into such a toxic environment with my mother. She was either putting me down for not trying hard enough or using me as her 'counsellor' to relieve herself of her 'problems' – eg her non-acceptance of Rupert being with Clare, her frustration of Damian not pulling his weight in the office and the strain of looking after Nan.

However, I was so emotionally weak and my mindset was screwed up (I hated myself). I felt more comfortable with the life I knew at home than taking a chance and living on campus. I was scared people would not accept me and would reject me.

I wish I had been stronger, taken a chance and stayed living on campus.

It's true to say my analytical mind (having to do well at university rather than being relaxed and enjoying myself) hadn't helped matters with Andrea. In reality, Andrea was a bit young and naïve, she wasn't interested in computers. She just wasn't the right person to help me at university.

After half term, once Andrea had left, in a way things got a little easier because she wasn't around anymore. On the other hand, I still felt extremely guilty – I thought I had failed with Andrea.

University was physically difficult. I didn't have a scribe in my lectures, so I photocopied someone else's handwritten notes. Watts Building had six floors and two lifts. Walking (and carrying my rucksack) around the place on my own was difficult. I didn't go to the canteen in the building opposite because it was too much hard work. Therefore, I just went to the little coffee and snack bar on the third floor in Watts and I became even more withdrawn.

I managed without another helper at university until the Christmas holidays.

I found another way of beating myself up. I started to compare myself to people who I thought were better than me. I compared myself to the two guys on my course who appeared to be superior to everybody else. This made me think I was useless and made me feel physically sick.

Comparing myself to other people was something I did in everyday life – and I continued to do so for the next five years, until 2001.

My vomiting at home became like a drug habit. The more times I threw up, the less stress release I got from doing so each time – therefore, I began vomiting more and more. I became caught in a vicious circle.

Throwing up became my coping mechanism. It was something I did, pretty much every day for the next sixteen years.

I would become so stressed, or feel like I had done something wrong, that the only way I knew how to feel better was by being sick, it wasn't unusual for me to throw up three times a day.

Over the years, only a few people knew about my vomiting – and some of them suggested I had bulimia. I wasn't bulimic. Being a person who doesn't tend to show negative emotions outwardly, vomiting was the only way I knew how to release stress and tension.

Throwing up was something I did mainly at home but I didn't keep it confined to vomiting in the toilet. A lot of time I was sick in the kitchen sink. Often however, I wouldn't get to the sink fast enough and my aim wasn't that good. Consequently I would throw up half in the sink and down the kitchen cupboards, on the floor. Having to clean it up wasn't very pleasant.

When I became stressed and felt sick when I was out somewhere, I would either wait until I got home, or vomit in the toilet or outside somewhere, out of sight. Over the two years I was at university, I only threw up on a couple of occasions there – in the toilet.

It's something I kept hidden and usually did when nobody else was around. The only people who really knew about it were Mum and Clare.

Mum's way of dealing with it was to pretend it wasn't happening by leaving me to it. Sometimes she stressed me out so much that I started convulsing (as if I was about to vomit) on front of her. At which point she shouted at me, "Stop it... don't do that... you're just indulging yourself..." The only effect shouting at me to stop it had was to make me think that I was even more useless and worthless, which made me throw up.

Clare was much more sympathetic. However, as Clare and I got on well, I normally didn't become stressed by her so I rarely was sick in front of her.

Writing about it now (in 2013) feels strange because, it was only in 2010, after learning about human behaviour and how the mind works, that I became aware and understood all of my negative thoughts (feeling I was worthless, useless and inadequate etc).

Up until that point, all my negative thoughts about myself were so subconscious I didn't know what they were. I spent years trying to work out why I was throwing up but I didn't realise why I was vomiting. Therefore, I accepted that vomiting was just something I did.

Having thrown up for so many years up until late 2010, today, I really appreciate not feeling sick.

Shortly after I moved back home from university campus, it felt like my confidence had hit rock bottom and I became even more isolated. It caused Mum to often have a go at me about something else – me not going out much. It didn't help matters.

I still went out with my cousins at the weekends and Keith and I often went to the cinema during the week. I also went over to Damian and Camille's place frequently, who had now bought and moved into a basement flat in Hove.

There was a girl called Amelia who I often saw around Watts building at university. She wore colourful clothes and seemed like a nice person – but I only had the confidence to say hello to her and ask her how she was.

At the start of the Christmas holidays back in December 1994, John Potts (JP), my new CSV university helper from Windsor, came to visit me at home with his parents. JP helped me at university for six months until the summer break. We became good friends and he was excellent at helping me on my course.

As he was ten months older than me, he had already obtained a BSc 1st in Finance. My HND course was like a walk in the park for JP! He was brilliant at going through matrices and other maths with me that I didn't quite understand at first.

JP became a family friend and often socialised with my cousins and I. He rented a room in a house opposite the university.

It was obvious that JP was exceptionally bright and dynamic and was going to do really well in life. Hence, I compared myself to him and felt I was far inferior. When we went to the canteen at university and I ate a meal including a pudding with custard, I often felt sick afterwards.

Now, it's ironic because I know JP finds me inspirational.

After helping me at university, JP went on to achieve a Masters degree, before getting a planning job with British Airways at Heathrow. His job involved planning how BA could maximise the usage of their aircrafts. At the time JP was living in Hounslow and every so often, either he came to see me or I went to see him.

Like me, JP is one of a handful of people I know who is both a people-person and an analytical person. It is rare for someone to have both of these personality traits.

In 2003, after travelling the world for twelve months, having got bored of the London rat race, JP moved to Ecuador. It didn't take him long to learn Spanish and to open up his own travel agency – Happy Gringo. Having just had a look at the website, the company now has twenty-three employees. I knew JP would do well in life. Thank you for inspiring me JP.

In 1995 I really got into listening to a new station called Talk Radio UK. Up until that point I had only listened to music radio. I enjoyed hearing something different and liked its current affairs content that Scott Chisholm, the mid-morning presenter, covered well.

Also entertaining were, as some people referred to them, 'shock-jocks', Tommy Boyd, Nick Abbot and late night presenter Caesar the Geezer. I found them creative and funny. I remembered Tommy Boyd from the mid-eighties, when he did a Sunday evening phone-in show on Southern Sound.

Another funny person on Talk Radio was solicitor Gary Jacobs, who did a legal advice phone-in show at the weekend. I recall hearing the following exchange, which made me laugh.

Caller: "My next door neighbour wants to build a wall between his house and my house, can he do it?"

Gary Jacobs: (Without hesitation) "I don't know, is he a bricklayer?"

Over the summer of 1995 I went on my first solo long distance holiday – it was a blast! I went to see my friend Jake in Los Angles (who I met at Club Med in the Bahamas).

As it was the first time I was travelling long distance on my own, I bought a cheap ticket, direct flight from Heathrow to LAX, on Virgin Atlantic (and got upgraded to business class for free!).

I've always been good at finding cheap flights and then getting the price down even more. At the time I used Teletext to get the phone numbers of about ten different travel agents. After phoning up a few of them, I established which flight and the dates I wanted to travel on. Afterwards I phoned all of the other travel agents to get a quote for the flights I wanted. I then phoned back the three agents with the cheapest quotes and, politely, haggled with them by playing one against the other. It really worked and it was good fun!

I phoned Clare to tell her I was going to see Jake in LA. She was excited for me and asked which airline I was flying with. I knew that this was going to cause me difficulty (hearing or saying a word which has a sexual connotation, due to my friendship with Nathan). I became embarrassed and breathless, saying 'Virgin', which I then beat myself up over the next few hours, for getting embarrassed.

There is an art, I have found, to getting upgraded on a plane – and there are several opportunities for trying to do so. The best time to ask is at the airport check-in desk because they allocate you a seat on your boarding pass.

The conversation with the check-in clerk goes something like this:

Me: "Hello, how are you doing today?"

(Wait for them to respond)

Me: "Good, excellent."

(Create a little bit of small talk)

Me: "I wonder if you can help me?"

(Wait for them to respond)

Me: Thank you."

Me: "I'm going on a long flight today and my knees and hamstring become really stiff when I sit with my legs bent. Is there any possibility you could upgrade me?"

The key is to be very engaging, polite and gracious. Also very important is making eye contact and smiling a lot.

If they don't upgrade me at the check-in desk, I ask at the boarding gate desk. The second best person to ask is one of airhostesses, when I sit in my initial seat. They often reply, "If you bear with me until after we have taken off, I'll see what I can do."

More often than not, over the years, I have been upgraded.

Some of you reading this may think I'm using my CP to my advantage. Perhaps I am. However, having the extra legroom really does make a difference to my hamstrings. I also enjoy the challenge of getting a free upgrade!

I have never believed in lying in life. But I do believe that if you don't ask, you don't get.

Virgin were good, they upgraded me on the way to and from LA.

Jake was living in Hawaii (and still is) but over the summer of 1995 he visited his family and friends. The two weeks I spent in America that holiday was like a road trip around LA/California. Having not been to America before I thought it was awesome.

Jake had quite a big and wealthy family. I met so many nice people and we didn't stay with the same person/people for more than two nights. Some days we stayed in big houses in places like Malibu and Bel Air, other times I slept on people's couches. It was a bit full on but it added to the enjoyment of the holiday.

Jake is eight years older than me and, as I mentioned earlier, he can be a bit wild sometimes (or at least he was back then).

Never will I forget the two hour drive we did to Bakersfield, where we went white-water rafting. We went with Jimmy (Jake's school friend) and Jimmy's girlfriend. Jake and I went to pick them up – and had a swim in Jimmy's back garden pool before heading off to Bakersfield.

The journey to Bakersfield included a pitch-dark long and winding mountainous road. It was scary. I thought we were going to drive off the cliff. Luckily, we made it to Bakersfield alive and well! We stayed in a cheap motel before going to the white water rafting centre, the next morning.

We were going on a two-day excursion and camped overnight. There were nineteen people on our trip, consisting of two eight-man kayaks and a safety boat. Jake and I had the best seats – we sat at the front of the safety boat with Geoff at the helm, doing all the work.

Everybody else was in one of the kayaks and had an oar each to paddle the boat. They all said it was hard work! It wasn't for Jake and I! We had an awesome time.

Before heading out on the River Kern on day one the organisers told me the river contained weeds and branches. They advised me if we capsized, to lift my feet and legs up to not get them caught in the undergrowth. I also had to sign a waiver in case I drowned!

The first day involved going through Class 2 and Class 3 rapids, which was exciting. However, on the second day we went through lots of Class 4 rapids. Sitting at the front of the boat became really scary (and exhilarating)!

All we could see ahead of us was the raging river of white-water. I kept thinking *we're never going to get through that...* It felt like we kept going down cliff faces of white water. It made my heart beat like the clappers. Jake was good, he kept holding onto my life jacket. If I was going into the river, he was coming in with me (or vice versa)! Thankfully, Geoff was very experienced at manoeuvring through the wild torrents and we didn't capsize.

I'm not sure if white water rafting is the most exhilarating I've done in life (so far), or whether it was skiing in Aspen.

My holiday to the west coast of America that year was the first of several adventures I've been on around the world. Whenever I've travelled somewhere, I've seen it as a real adventure and lived more in the moment. I've met a lot of people around the world who are amazed that I go travelling on my own. I don't see it as a big deal because I get assistance at airports.

The downside of travelling on my own is not having my car. Therefore, I rely on my wheelchair, which is difficult for me to push myself in – and sitting in it for long periods tightens up my hamstrings. Also, over the years I've come to not like going on holiday on my own. I would much rather have someone to go with.

My flight from LAX back to Heathrow left in the evening. However, early that afternoon, Jake had an appointment to go to. Hence, we put my suitcase in a locker at the airport and Jake dropped me off at Venice Beach, in time to make his appointment.

Venice Beach is an area with lots of market stalls and bars. I had a fun afternoon talking to people there. I also bought about ten t-shirts (to give to my family) from one of the market stalls, before getting a taxi to the airport.

One of the t-shirts I got there is my Bob Marley t-shirt, which I still have today. It's a white t-shirt with Bob Marley's face covering the front of it. Whenever I wear it people always comment what a cool t-shirt it is!

Musically, I think Bob Marley is in a league of his own.

Back at home, later that summer, Clare and Rupert came to stay with us for a few days – and announced that Clare was pregnant. It was a bit of a surprise to me but not totally unexpected, Clare was twenty-three and had been with Rupert for about four years. It was more of a shock to Mum due to her dislike and disapproval of Rupert. It created a bit of an awkward situation when they broke the news. Mum went on about it to me, in her unaccepting rants, once Clare and Rupert had gone back to Coventry.

Returning to university in September, my new CSV helper for that term was Ed. He was slightly younger than me but he was responsible and did the job well. He joined the local choir and I remember going to St Peter's Church, just before the end of term, to see (and hear) Ed sing. He was good.

In early 1996, Clare gave birth to Scott. Mum went up to stay with them first, before I picked Dad up from Gatwick and drove to Coventry (it felt like a reversal of roles!). I was driving on the motorway when I saw something spooky happen in my rear-view mirror – the boot of my car suddenly came wide open! I pulled onto the hard shoulder and Dad shut it – properly this time!

We stayed with Clare and Rupert (who were living in a crappy first floor flat) for a couple of days. It was really good seeing Scott.

Once the baby was born, Mum was a little more relaxed and Clare and Scott regularly came home to stay for a few days. I became no stranger to holding Scott in my arms – I liked my new role as an uncle. Mum was good with Scott too.

At university I had a new helper called Ralph. He was a local guy in his thirties who Trish had found for me. Ralph did the job and we got on okay – but he didn't totally respect me and was cocky. I think he saw helping me out as an easy way of making a few quid.

Shortly before the end of term, Ralph mentioned that he was thinking about going camping with a mate of his for four days at Easter, at the end of April.

A place that I had heard about and looked into was the Orthotic Research & Locomotor Assessment Unit (ORLAU) in Oswestry, Shropshire, where there is a gait analysis laboratory.

Gait analysis is used to assess and treat people who have walking difficulties. It is a study of human motion by measuring the body's mechanics and the activity of the muscles.

At the time, I think ORLAU was the only place in the UK who did gait analysis. I was still wearing a calliper below my knee on my left leg and dragging my foot. I asked Alison Smith to refer me for an assessment.

Mum and I spent two days at ORLAU over the Easter holidays. It was a distance of two hundred and fifty miles from home and we shared the driving.

I had the gait analysis on the first day and it seemed very high-tech. It involved me walking up and down a little 'runway' wearing just a pair of shorts and a load of electrodes on my body, with cameras filming me from every angle. They taped up the sides of my shorts so that they could film my hips. I felt like I was a model in a skimpy pair of shorts walking up and down a catwalk!

The second day was with the director of ORLAU, Professor John Patrick. He was a well-spoken, grey haired man in his fifties, with good people skills. It was obvious that he knew what he was doing and was a highly experienced surgeon. Mr Patrick had examined my performance as a model and told me to not give up my day job! Joking aside, he said the gait analysis had shown that I use four times the amount of energy walking of an average person, and he recommended performing an operation on my left foot to straighten it and stop me from dragging it. My analytical side kicked in then and I asked a load of questions.

Mr Patrick said that at twenty-two I was slightly old for the operation (because my body was fully grown), but he didn't perceive any problems. The operation entailed breaking three bones and resetting them. My foot would be in plaster for three or four months, during which time I wouldn't be able to walk.

I wanted to know what the reduction in my energy consumption would be as a result of having the surgery, but Mr Patrick said it wasn't possible for him to make such a prediction. However, he was obviously the person to perform the operation – which we scheduled for September.

One thing Mum and I noticed in Oswestry was how all of the people we met were so open and friendly. Over the next few years I came to think, in general, northerners are much more friendly and helpful than people from the south-east of England.

I find this also applies to black people. When it came to doing group assignments at university, I tended to work with David and Robert, the two black guys on my course, because I got on with them far better than some of the other people.

In late April, Ralph was off sick for, initially, a couple days, which he then extended to four days. All of my lectures and exams were over by then. All I had left to do at university was a final project, that I had well under control and didn't need Ralph's help with. Therefore, I thanked him for all of his help and told him I didn't need him anymore. Had I felt that Ralph was being honest with me I wouldn't have got rid of him.

In May, Damian introduced me to a guy he knew called Ray, who had been to see Damian and his band perform at local pubs and clubs. At the time Ray was running Festival FM – a temporary RSL (Restricted Service Licence) radio station, which was on air for the duration for the Brighton Fringe Festival in 1996. When Ray invited Damian into the station for an interview about his band, Damian mentioned that I was really interested in getting into radio and Ray suggested that Damian bring me along with him.

Meeting Ray was a defining event. After we chatted for a few minutes he could see how eager I was to get into radio. Ray said that he was heading a bid, and was one of the applicants, to win the licence to run a full-time radio station in Brighton.

Ray said that in early 1997 he would be opening an office and working full-time with a small team of volunteers, to promote and gain support for his radio licence bid application. Ray invited me along and said I would be welcome to help out. I thought: *There's going to be a new radio station in Brighton and this is my chance.*

In completing my HND at university I achieved a distinction or merit in every module. Although I didn't get as many distinctions as I did at college, I was slightly surprised that I had done so well. I hadn't enjoyed university and found it really tough; thinking I was worthless and useless, always comparing myself to others and feeling I was inadequate. Also, I hadn't liked the need to have a scribe and helper in lectures.

With hindsight, had I been in a good frame of mind, the HND at Chichester College would have been far easier for me to do.

My graduation ceremony was at the Brighton Centre in May. Clare, Scott, Mum, Liz and Mandy came to it. I remember queuing up, in my graduation gown and hat, with the people on my course to go up on stage, one by one. After collecting my certificate I became self-conscious at the whole audience looking at me and applauding. I was scared I was going fall down the steps walking off the stage! It made me walk really slowly and I was fine.

After the meal at the Brighton Centre, we all went across the road onto the promenade. It was a sunny day and I felt hot in my graduation attire. People wanted to take photos of me leaning against the railings, with the beach and sea in the background. Although I wasn't holding onto my crutches I had my arms through the hoops of them, which was helping me to balance myself. At which point Mum came up, took the crutches from my arms and said, "You don't need these, they'll spoil the photos."

It's not the cleverest thing my mother has ever done and I felt like screaming at her. However, there were loads of people around and I didn't want to create a scene – so I said nothing.

By taking my crutches off of me, it put my upper-legs and knees under enormous strain and I nearly fell over. Then, Clare gave me Scott to hold!

Somewhere is the photo of me holding Scott, with a sort of grin on my face, trying desperately hard not to fall over. My grin was out of pain – not pleasure.

Mum wanted me to go on and do a degree at university. She wanted me to have an 'ology'. An HND was good enough for me and I was pleased to have got university over and done with. My abiding memory of the place is of feeling sick most of the time I was there.

I was now absolutely determined to work in radio.

Chapter 8

At the end of June 1996, it was time to get a new Motability car. I went for another Vauxhall Astra, this time in turquoise.

A few days after I got my new Astra I went to a reunion for people who were part of Barley at secondary school. As I drove to my old school, I felt proud of my new car because I thought I would be one of the few people at the reunion who was able to drive there.

I didn't know who to expect to see at the reunion. I thought all of my school friends who had Muscular Dystrophy (MD) would have died years earlier. It's a very good thing I went because Martin was at the reunion (my friend with MD who I had met in April 1984, at middle school). I was absolutely elated to see Martin again. I lost touch with him when I went to boarding school in 1988.

What's more, Martin was there with Janet, his heavily pregnant wife, who he had recently married. For someone who was about to turn twenty-two, Martin was defying the odds for someone with MD to still be alive. Although, he had lost a lot of strength, since I had last seen him, he seemed well. Martin said he was living in a residential home near Chichester and I went to see him the following weekend.

Another person I swapped phone numbers with at the school reunion was Monica, a girl with Spina Bifida, who I used to go horse riding with on Tuesday afternoons.

When I arrived at Martin's home a couple of days later, the people who worked there said, "Martin's at the pub around the corner. He said to tell you to go and join him." They explained where the pub was and I drove there.

As I walked into the pub, I saw Martin, sitting with Janet and a number of other people drinking JD and cokes. In a few minutes it became obvious that Martin was a fun guy and he had a lot of life left in him. We stayed at the pub for a while before going back to his home.

Martin went back home in his electric wheelchair with a few people, whilst I drove with Janet because I didn't know how to get back there.

There were three other disabled guys living in Martin's home who coincidentally I knew from boarding school. The home was staffed with five or six CSVs (Community Service Volunteers). Janet was one of them but, with her baby coming in September, she was due to stop working shortly. The CSVs lived upstairs in the home and worked shifts to provide 24 hour care for the four disabled guys.

Martin was so weak it was as if he was paralysed from the neck down. He just had enough strength in his left index finger to press a button the size of a Jaffa Cake, to control his electric wheelchair. He used another button, when he was in bed, which connected to infrared devices. Using one button, Martin controlled his TV, video, hifi, PC etc. He was very good at art and drawing on his computer. When he was at home Martin wore an oxygen mask over his nose (which was connected to a battery pack). His lungs almost didn't work anymore.

There was nothing wrong with Martin's mind. He was as sharp as anyone – and he had an absolute will to live. He nearly always seemed so positive and in good spirits (mostly Jack Daniels!). Martin really inspired me.

Over the next few months and years I went to see Martin every three or four weeks. We often went to the pub together and got drunk! I went in my wheelchair but I didn't have to push myself – I just held onto the side of Martin's wheelchair. I rarely used my wheelchair but I felt comfortable using it to go to the pub with Martin.

Martin drank JD and Coke and I drank vodka-oranges. He drank from a glass and a straw that I held up to his mouth. We had a real laugh and liked the same music; Manic Street Preachers, Britpop and Nirvana.

His arms laid on the armrests of his wheelchair and sometimes Martin asked me something like, "Could you move my right arm back a bit." His arms were like matchsticks.

When I went to see Martin and got drunk, I either slept the night on a mattress on the floor of his room, or upstairs in the volunteers' lounge.

One night when I was sleeping in his room, Martin developed serious trouble breathing so the person on night duty called an ambulance. I was really scared he wasn't going to make it through the night – but Martin was a fighter and he pulled through.

On other occasions (not after getting drunk with me) he went into hospital with a chest infection. He twice came back to life after the hospital declared him clinically dead!

Shortly after the school reunion in July, Monica and I loosely went out for about three weeks and we saw each other most days during that time. I found her slightly immature and we had nothing in common. As I had bought tickets to see Bryan Adams at Wembley, who Monica really wanted to see, I took her to the concert, before I ended things shortly afterwards. I did feel sorry for Monica because she really liked me. I don't like hurting people.

Mum and I weren't getting on well. She always wanted to know where I was going, what I was doing, who I was going to see etc. I felt like I had absolutely no space. It was suffocating.

In early August, we went on a family holiday to South Africa and Mozambique. Mum and I were getting on so badly that I didn't know whether to go on the holiday or to stay at home and have a two week break from her.

Thinking it would be foolish of me not to go on such a holiday, I made the decision on the night before we left. Not all of the family went – only Damian and Camille, Keith and his girlfriend, Mum, Liz, john and I.

It was a real eye-opener. We flew to Johannesburg, where we stayed for three days. All of the taxi drivers in Johannesburg had one or two guns in the boot of their cars, which felt daunting. The culture there seemed to be about survival of the fittest.

We travelled to Mozambique by minibus and went round the country for ten days. Although I've never been a materialistic person, it still gave me another perspective on life. Seeing the abject poverty and the devastation caused by the civil war; people living in mud huts or in a shell of a building; people walking for miles every day just to get water, or scrambling around for leftover food.

It made me think, *as long as you've got somewhere to live, enough to eat and someone to share your life with, nothing else really matters.*

It's not uncommon for the poorest people in the world to be the most generous and welcoming people on earth. They understand how precious life is.

Writing about it now, I feel like going to find a sweet African woman to marry, love and to take care of.

I feel my monthly £15 donation to Action Aid since the age of twelve is insignificant. I feel like I should be doing much more to help people in life.

Going on to write about something else in my book feels odd because, without realising it, I've just outlined the two things I really care about in life.

In mid-September, I had the operation on my left foot in Oswestry. I remember coming round/waking up after the surgery. It felt like a piece of lead was on my foot and it was very painful. This is where the Morphine came in!

During the operation they had put 'a line' into my arm (I'm not sure if that's the correct medical term), so that I could inject myself with Morphine. I loved it! Every few minutes I could press a button which released a bit more Morphine into my body. It was excellent – it relieved the pain I was in and made me feel slightly lightheaded!

I don't advocate the use of drugs but Morphine is great in small doses. Where can I get some now? I need a fix!

The day after the operation I was out of bed and in my wheelchair. The surgery had disturbed the blood circulation in my foot. Hence, I had to keep my foot elevated while I was in plaster. When it wasn't raised my foot became really heavy within a few minutes.

I went around in my wheelchair with my left leg and foot straight out in front of me, resting on a black padded plank of wood. This reduced the amount of thrust I had in my arms to push myself around – but I managed to do so slowly.

With Oswestry being on the north Welsh border, the hospital was full of young Welsh female nurses – and I loved it! I was going around cracking jokes, making them laugh. They were lovely.

The nurses kept chatting amongst themselves about going to 'Abba'. I couldn't work out what on earth they meant. At first I thought they were excited about going to see an ABBA tribute group. I had to ask them what they were referring to. They told me that Abba was short for Aberystwyth (where they were going on holiday)!

The other reason I loved being in hospital was because Mum wasn't there and I didn't have any stress. It was like being on holiday and there were always people to chat with. I stayed in hospital for as long as I could. I knew that being confined to a wheelchair at home with Mum was going to be a nightmare.

Mr Patrick came to see me every day. I was fine but became completely paranoid. I wasn't meant to put weight on my foot. Going around in my wheelchair, with my foot out in front of me, it was easy to accidently knock it against something. Every time I knocked it slightly, I thought I had damaged my foot and it wouldn't heal properly. Mr Patrick told me not to let it worry me but to be careful.

Now that I knew Mr Patrick a little more I asked him if he would mind me calling him John. He replied, "If you would like to do so," but it didn't make me feel comfortable – so I continued to call him Mr Patrick!

About a week after my operation, the plaster of Paris was taken off, my foot was X-rayed and a lighter, yellowy plaster was put on it. The X-ray revealed I had a metal staple hoop in my foot.

After the gait analysis at Easter, when I asked Mr Patrick what the operation involved, he didn't say he was going to put a piece of metal in my foot. What happens if it becomes rusty? It's not like I can open up my foot and spray some WD40 on it!

I managed to stay in hospital for three weeks.

With Coventry not that far from Oswestry, Clare came (with Scott) to pick me up. It was always nice to see Scott. We went back to Clare's flat and Clare and Rupert carried me up the stairs. Mum came to get me the same day.

Life at home in my wheelchair was a nightmare. I wasn't even able to go to the toilet standing up. Instead I urinated into one of those plastic bottles that some disabled people use – which I didn't like much. It felt more acceptable to use a bottle in hospital than at home.

Although Mum went into the office most days, I was dependent on her for some things. It was horrible because she had more power over me. Inevitably, it caused even more arguments (than the usual ones) and I found it very stressful because I couldn't get away. I couldn't escape. My three week break from vomiting was over.

Two weeks after coming out of hospital, I could suddenly move my foot slightly in the plaster. My analytical mind started to panic, thinking, *I'm not meant to do that!* It caused me to phone ORLAU a couple of times, who told me to relax and that it was normal. Thinking about it now, it's obvious why I could move my foot slightly – it had lost a bit of weight being in plaster.

Clare came to stay for a while which was nice. Due to me being in my wheelchair the whole time it caused my right hamstring to really tighten up. Somehow, I came across Sally Gunnell's physiotherapist, who came to see me.

I don't remember her name but she was very good. I hadn't come across her technique of stretching hamstrings before. With me lying on my front, on the sofa, she stood on the sofa and put the heel of one of her feet on my hamstring and pressed down on it. It proved to be effective. She also had a baby boy who was the same age as Scott.

I did go out with my cousins while in plaster. Somewhere odd that we went to was to watch a local amateur boxing match. It was odd because it's not something I would normally go to see.

I've always thought boxing is a barbaric sport because I don't see the point of two people trying to knock each other out. At least it got me out of the house.

A week before Christmas 1996, Damian and I went to Oswestry. Before we left home Mr Patrick told me that they were going to remove the plaster, X-ray my foot and put another plaster on it for about another month.

When we got there – and after they had taken off the plaster (with the dreaded circular saw) and my foot had been X-rayed – Mr Patrick announced, "I'm very pleased to say your foot has healed extremely well and is absolutely fine. You can go home now!"

As I was expecting to be in plaster for another month or so, it completely threw me.

Me: "I can't go home like this. I can't walk yet!"

Mr Patrick: "You'll just have to be patient and wait until the New Year. I will ensure you get the rehabilitation physio you need at your local hospital."

I was extremely thankful and grateful. I really respect Mr Patrick.

Knowing how paranoid I was about my foot not healing properly, Mr Patrick had fooled me into believing I needed to be in plaster for longer! Obviously he was also playing it safe, depending on the X-ray.

The funny thing was, I didn't have the shoe for my left foot – so Damian and I had to go into Oswestry to buy a pair of shoes!

It felt a bit odd spending Christmas unable to walk. At least with my foot out of plaster, my blood circulation soon got back to normal and I didn't need to keep my foot elevated anymore.

I wasted no time chasing up my physio rehab on 2 January 1997. I wanted to learn to walk again and get back to full strength as quickly as possible. I had plans!

Prior to having the operation, I had a lot of stamina, could walk up to fifty yards or so and had no problems walking up and down stairs.

The first couple of physio sessions I had felt very strange because I could only manage to walk a short distance in the parallel bars, before becoming out of breath. It frustrated me and I thought, *I'm never going to back to normal at this rate.* But I knew I was going to make a full recovery.

Thankfully, I was going to the main physio department at my local hospital – and not the neurological one I went to years earlier.

I had physio two to three times a week. Within the second week I started walking short distances with my crutches. This was a big step because I then started walking around at home again.

The way I have always walked up stairs is by going up one step at a time – with my left foot first – and putting weight on it to walk up the step with my right foot. However, the first time I tried to walk up a step in my physio rehab I thought I couldn't do it.

I was scared to put so much weight on my left foot – I thought doing so would break it! My foot still felt tender – or rather, my mind thought it was. I was so scared of hurting my left foot that I tried walking up the steps using my right foot first. However, with my right foot being the weaker one of the two, it took more energy and I was making life more difficult for myself. It was just another case of feeling the fear and doing it anyway.

Once I had overcome the obstacle in my mind and I started walking up steps with my left foot first, I felt an enormous sense of achievement and there was no stopping me!

It was absolutely vital that I learnt to manage stairs again.

The first thing I did once I could walk a short distance and drive my car again, was go to see Martin and Janet. In September Janet had given birth to Ben and I hadn't seen their new baby yet. It was great seeing Ben and, fortunately, he hadn't inherited the defective gene which causes MD. I started to go and see them every few weeks again.

As Janet had stopped working at Martin's residential home prior to giving birth, she was now living (with Ben) in a council house nearby. Martin and Janet wanted to move into a house together. It took about three years to happen because they went through a lot of bureaucracy to obtain a suitable property and arrange around the clock carers for Martin.

In the end, I only had six or seven weeks of physio rehab and I was pleased with how quickly I had recovered. I was walking with my left foot much straighter and virtually wasn't dragging it anymore. What's more, I was no longer wearing a calliper on my leg. As I've said before, when I think of the long-term gain from having an operation, I dismiss the short-term pain and inconvenience I went through.

At the end of the previous chapter I said I was determined to work in radio. My eagerness to start working with Ray, and be part of his bid team for the Brighton radio licence, was the reason I wanted to quickly learn to walk again (as opposed to learn to walk quickly again!).

The office they were working from was on the main Lewes Road in Brighton, which didn't have any off-road parking. Therefore, I needed to be able to walk the relatively short distance from where I parked my car. Also, they were working in a basement office, hence, I needed to be able to walk up and down a flight of stairs!

I started working with New Wave Broadcasting (the company Ray formed for the Radio licence) in the last week of February. The place always seemed to be a hive of activity and it was good fun to be a part of it.

Alongside a team of people, Ray had already submitted New Wave's bid to run the full-time radio station in Brighton. There were three or four other bidders going for the licence, which the Radio Authority were due to award in the summer. As New Wave seemed to be the only bidders who were doing something to gain support after submitting their licence application, there was a great atmosphere of anticipation in the office.

Ray was working full-time on the bid and was in the office every day promoting their radio station (called Passion). Adrian, Barry and Ted were also part of the bid and came into the office most days. The office also contained two fairly primitive radio studios and there were a load of other volunteers, who came in and out every day, helping in the office and using the studios.

Two volunteers I remember the most were Alison Hulme (who was about my age) and sixteen-year-old Seth.

It was good being around so many like-minded people. I immediately got on well with Ray and everyone and I went into the office virtually every day, cracking jokes and helping Ray with documentation. I recall drafting a letter to The Prodigy's Keith Flint who was one of New Wave's supporters.

Ray and I became good friends and I learnt that in 1985, Ray and Ted set up Worthing Hospital Radio - and they ran a number of Brighton RSL stations in the nineties. Ray had been working and lobbying for a full-time radio station in Brighton for the past two years.

As well as helping in the office, I took the opportunity to gain experience using the equipment in the radio studios.

I should probably mention that my passion for working in radio has always been about working behind the scenes. I love pushing buttons and making things happen. I'm a great button pusher! When it comes to working in a radio studio I am completely self-taught. I've never had the desire to be a radio presenter.

It is also worth pointing out that Ted is the person I met when I joined hospital radio in 1993, who said to me, "There's no point in me teaching you how to use the studio because you're never going to be a radio presenter."

The impression I got from Ted was that he was bemused to see me at New Wave but we got on okay, as I had little to do with him there.

It's funny, I wouldn't describe myself as a creative person but when it comes to radio I am. The first thing I made was an advert for a fictitious taxi firm (called X-Cabs). After I had written the ad, I asked Alison Hulme to voice it for me. Then, using editing software on my PC at home, I made a thirty second music bed, from the song 'Get the Funk Out' by Extreme.

A (music) bed is a piece of instrumental music (without any singing on it), which a radio presenter talks over. Music beds are also often used in radio adverts (ie the background music of an advert).

Once I had made the music bed, I mixed it with the recording of Alison's voice – it was easy and my ad sounded really good!

Alison went on to do well working in radio, later winning awards. I've just Googled her, after sixteen years – I see she's got a PhD and is a university lecturer!

After making my ad, I was more adventurous and had the idea of a thirty-minute programme containing music and news items. First, I had to get some news material so I recorded some items from my local BBC radio station.

Purely by chance, I picked a good day for news. It was on a day leading up to the second round of the Conservative leadership election in 1997. I obtained a report on the upcoming leadership election from Mark Sanders and a clip from each of the three candidates – Ken Clarke, William Hague and John Redwood (aka Spock from *Star Trek*).

The BBC station also did a feature on a car-free day and I got a forty-five second report on it.

I chose four songs. Two of them were 'Cars' by Gary Numan and 'Somewhere' by Efua – a fun and quirky track I heard Simon Bates championing on Radio 1 in 1993. He predicted the single would get to number 1. It only reached number 42!

In sequencing the running order, I intertwined the news items between the songs, and wrote an informative script to introduce each song, news clip and report. I put the X-Cabs ad in the middle of the programme. All I needed was someone to record all of the links. Barry kindly pre-recorded them for me. He must have done nine or ten links.

On a CD of music beds at New Wave I found the bed that Scott Chisholm was using on Talk Radio. As I liked the bed, I decided to use it at the start and end of my programme – and played Barry's first and last link over it.

When I had edited all of the individual speech elements I was ready to put the whole show together. However, I was a bit nervous! I knew if I made a mistake at any point I would have to start the whole show again.

Having thought about it for a few days, I waited until after six o'clock one evening (when most people had gone home), and I went for it.

Being completely focussed on what I was doing, I made no errors and did the programme on the first take. The show was twenty-seven minutes long. I was really pleased with what I had created.

Barry had done a link to introduce the report on the carfree day. As the report was forty-five seconds long and the intro on 'Cars' by Gary Numan is thirty seconds, I started the song fifteen seconds into the report – so that the vocals in the song kicked in when the report ended. I back-timed it perfectly and it sounded slick. (All these years later I don't remember the exact timings! I'm using these figures to illustrate back-timing).

I did the show using two mini disc players, two CD players and a cart machine. On one mini disc were Barry's links, on the other were all of the news items. While one CD was playing I cued-up the other one with the next song. It was easy in the end.

It was easy because I planned it very well and was fully focussed but, above all, I *knew* that I could do it. It started out as an idea I had.

Using the twenty-seven minute recording of the show, I made an edited version of it by cutting out the middle part of each song, and put both versions of the show onto a number of cassette tapes.

I then thought of trying to get some work experience at Spirit FM in Chichester and sent them a letter and a copy of my tape. After chasing them up a couple of times by phone, they offered me a week's work experience! In organising my work experience, Bernard Allen commented that he was extremely impressed with my tape.

I also sent my tape to Southern FM, but in all the years I contacted them, they never seemed interested in me.

Launched in 1996, Spirit was a small station. At the time when I did my work experience (in June 1997), each of the weekday presenters worked full-time there, which consisted of presenting a daily four hour show and a desk-based role in the office. The station is in a small-ish two storey building with an office on the ground floor and a wide staircase up to the studios and newsroom.

My work experience at Spirit was great fun. Ian Crouch (Crouchie) was the person who scheduled the music, which I did a bit of. As well as doing some ad trafficking (scheduling) and editing, I also sat in the studio with the drivetime presenter who, ironically, came to work on his bicycle!

During the day all of the songs were played from CDs and there was a computer play-out system (Audio Vault) for the jingles and adverts. It was the first radio play-out system I had come across.

As 'I Wanna Be the Only One' by Eternal/BeBe Winans was in the charts, it always reminds me of my week's work experience at Spirit.

However, I only did four days of work experience at the station because on the Thursday of that week was the big announcement from the Radio Authority, about who was going to be awarded the Brighton licence.

I will never forget that day. In the morning the New Wave office was buzzing and crammed with people. There was an air of excitement and of slight tension. Ray's wife and two little boys were there – as were Meridian TV News. Everyone was waiting for the phone call from the Radio Authority.

Then at about 11.30 am it came. The phone rang – everyone became a bit more excited – as Ray answered the phone, everyone hushed. Within five to ten seconds the excitement turned into devastation, The Radio Authority was phoning to inform New Wave that they had awarded the Brighton radio licence to one of the other contenders.

Nobody in the office could believe it. It made some people cry. Ray and his team had devoted so much of their time and energy campaigning for a radio station in Brighton and New Wave had gained a lot of support for its bid. It turned into a fairy sombre afternoon. Ray felt he had let everybody down.

The next day, driving to Chichester for my last day of work experience at Spirit, I felt a bit strange. Obviously, New Wave not winning the licence was a big blow but I didn't let the disappointment diminish my determination to work in radio.

That Friday at Spirit was the start of a silver lining for me. Kevin Dyball, the Programme Controller, who also presented the breakfast show, said that as from September they were going to need technical help on the Saturday afternoon sports show (which Kevin also presented) – and that I had the skills they needed! I felt delighted.

I've got my foot in the door at Spirit, I thought. *There's still going to be a new radio station in Brighton (called Surf) – I've just got to get my foot in the door with them as well.*

What's more, Ray and I were now good friends.

In July 1997 I went to visit my friend Jake, in Hawaii, for two weeks, who lives on an island called Maui. As I mentioned earlier in the book, whenever I go on holiday I see it as a great adventure and become more relaxed.

It took twenty hours and three plane rides to get there. It was an easy journey because I got assistance at every airport. The hardest part was sitting on planes for so long. I flew to San Francisco, onto Honolulu and then Maui. Although I got upgraded on the flights to San Francisco and Honolulu, it still gave me a numb bum!

Sitting in the front row of an old 100-seater plane to Maui, I noticed on the two front doors of the aircraft, in big red letters, was 'LEFT DOOR' and 'RIGHT DOOR'. It made me think, *this plane could fall apart at any moment!*

It was fun seeing Jake again and Maui was good. I met lots of people and went surfing (or rather, body-boarding) on the North Shore – where surfing competitions are held.

Jake asked me if I wanted to go skydiving. I consider myself as quite an adventurous person but after the accident I had with Rupert in Greece, where he tripped over my feet going parasailing, I thought the same might happen with skydiving – and I wasn't prepared to take the risk. It would have been a tandem skydive with an instructor. I think he might have tripped over my feet walking out of the plane, we would then end up freefalling in a spin and the instructor wouldn't be able to open the parachute!

I wouldn't mind going paragliding because it doesn't involve freefalling.

We went to Honolulu for a couple of days, staying with Jake's friends. I preferred Honolulu as it's more urban than Maui. There are two climates on Maui. One side of the island is dry and sandy, the other side is foresty and rainy. (On the whole, Hawaii is like California but even more relaxed). Jake lived in the jungle, renting a cabin the size of a postage stamp.

My friendship with Jake is a funny one. We go for years without speaking to each other – and then when I go and see him, we're like brothers. However, I found that I could only take him in small doses, of about a week.

I think it's because we have (or had) different realities. With Jake having, and being brought up by, a wealthy family, he didn't have to work and therefore he had an easy life. In 1997 he was doing a PhD in anthropology – because it interested him.

There's nothing wrong with the way Jake treated me but I found him to be extreme sometimes. His attitude seemed like, 'I've got my life and you've got yours. Get on with it...'

Where he lived, it took me a good five minutes to walk from his car to his cabin. When we came back from going out somewhere in the evening, we both got out of the car and he would say to me, "See you in about five minutes," and left me to find my way back to the cabin, through the forest and in the darkness of the night! I found it odd because people normally ask me if I need any help. The fact that he doesn't treat me any differently to anyone else is partly why we get on so well.

The other thing that I found strange, when I arrived in Maui, was that Jake didn't have any bedding for me. Therefore, I bought some there and left it with him when I left.

I decided to leave Hawaii a few days earlier than planned and spent the remaining time of my holiday in San Francisco. I managed to change my flight without a problem but was unable to find a hotel, before I left Maui. I thought, *I'll find a hotel when I get to San Francisco.*

Arriving at San Francisco airport at about 9.00 pm, I put my suitcase in an airport locker (and put a few clothes in my rucksack) and spent ages on the phone, trying to find a hotel room. Eventually finding one, I took an airport minibus which dropped people off at various hotels along the way. With me being the last person to be dropped off it got me wondering, *what is my hotel going to be like?*

It was after midnight when the minibus arrived at my abode and it didn't look good. It scared me to the point that I asked the driver, "Are you sure this is the right hotel?"

It was in a dark and grotty backstreet, which looked like a gangland drug dealer area! I checked into the small poky hotel a little nervously. It took me a while before I got to sleep that night. In the morning I wasted no time in checking out of the hotel and getting the hell out of that area.

After having a big breakfast in a diner (I love American diners), I found a much nicer hotel in a more central location. Then, wandering around the busy streets, I decided to go the famous square in San Francisco.

I started asking passers-by, "Excuse me, can you tell how to get to Times Square?" But they all looked at me a bit oddly and walked straight past me. I thought, *what's going on? I'm asking a perfectly reasonable question.* Until one guy said, "Don't you mean Union Square? Times Square is in New York!"

Me: "That's it! I'm not from round here..."

I told you I wasn't very good at remembering names or geography!

On the way to Union Square, one of my anti-tip bars fell off of my wheelchair! It was a problem because it held one of my crutches on the back of my wheelchair. I wondered how I was going to find someone who had an Allen key.

I was sitting in my wheelchair holding one of my sticks in between my legs and my anti-bar in my hand – in the middle of San Francisco. I started asking people, "Excuse me, please could you help me? I need to find someone who has got an Allen key to put this back on my wheelchair." It only took a few minutes to find someone.

After all, I was in America, where anything is possible!

San Francisco is a funny place because it's full of hills. It makes it either really easy or difficult when you're in a manual wheelchair – but people always helped me up the hills.

That evening, with my mind set on working in radio, I thought it would be fun to visit some radio stations the next day. I looked in the phone book and found there were six stations in one street. I went to all of them the following day.

The stations were on high floors in tall buildings. With my holiday confidence, I walked into each one saying, "Hello, I live in the UK and work as a radio studio producer. I wanted to come and say hello and see your set up." People were impressed and happy to show me around. I thought there was an outside chance that they would offer me a job!

In 2010 I read *Rich Dad Poor Dad* (the best book I've ever read). In it Robert Kiyosaki says 'If you go around telling people you're going to do something, you're more likely to achieve it.'

And that was my holiday adventure in 1997.

Elsewhere that year, Rupert's job in Coventry came to an end so he and Clare (and Scott) moved back to Shoreham. Initially they lived with us for a few weeks before they bought a house. The property they purchased was opposite ours, in the road behind our one. It meant our rear gardens backed onto each other and we put a gate in the fence for easy access.

It was really nice having Clare and Scott living nearby – and Clare was pregnant again.

As Nan had been living with us for a few years, to give Mum and I a break she moved in with Liz and John. Nan's Alzheimer's had noticeably deteriorated. It was a struggle to get her to eat anything. She often tried to offer her food to everyone else, saying, "Go on, you have it. I haven't touched it..."

All Nan wanted to do was go to see her father in Eric Street. With her asking to go and see him numerous times a day, it was a case of replying, "We can go tomorrow." Saying this prevented her from crying.

Things didn't improve much at home. Mum and I still argued a lot of the time. Tensions were building in the office and she would regularly come home from work and let out her frustrations by moaning at me; either by complaining about how Liz and John were letting Damian get away with doing little work, or about her dislike of Rupert – or about me being lazy and not going out much in the evenings. I used to think that she used me as her emotional punch-bag.

One thing Mum often used to do, while I was sitting on the green leather sofa watching TV, was to come into the lounge and rant at me for a few minutes. She knew she could do so because she knew that I was 'sunk' into the sofa and it was difficult for me to get up and leave the room.

With the sofa being low and soft it took me a couple of minutes and a lot of effort, pushing down on the sofa with my left hand and holding my stick with my right hand, to stand up.

When I got myself up or shouted back at her it just created more arguments. Hence, I often let her rants and ravings wash over me. When Mum felt she was losing an argument she would escape by going upstairs or into the back garden – or go over to Clare's house to moan about me. With Mum being a very influential and controlling person, she would get Clare on her side. It wasn't uncommon for the two of them to be having a go at me.

My daily chore was to unstack the dishwasher. It was quite hard carrying plates or pots and pans with one hand, while walking with just one stick – but I did it. I saw it as a few minutes of hard work. I wouldn't be surprised if it never crossed Mum's mind how much energy I used in unstacking the dishwasher. It seemed to her like just a little thing I did.

Writing about the very toxic relationship I had with my Mum, it surprises me, years later, that I just put up with it. The toxic relationship didn't do my mindset any good and I was emotionally very weak. It stressed me out and didn't make me feel good about myself. The only way I knew how to relieve the stress I was feeling was by vomiting.

On 1st May 1997, I stayed up most of night watching the general election unfold and felt euphoric when Tony Blair became prime minister. Eighteen years of Tory rule was over!

I received a surprising letter from Neil (the manic depressive), saying he didn't expect to die for many years and he had added me to his will. Mum received a similar letter from him.

My mate, Malc, found a girlfriend and moved from Croydon to somewhere up north with her. When Malc moved it didn't really bother me because I didn't see him that much. We only really used to go to the pub with Keith.

In August 1997, I went to see Ray at home on a sunny Sunday afternoon. I hadn't seen him since before I went on holiday to Hawaii and he still seemed disappointed about not winning the radio licence. He said he was going to talk to Surf about working for them – but he thought it would take a few months for the radio station to launch. In the meantime, Ray said he would need to find another job.

Ray is one of these people who has got a vast record collection and a dedicated music room with thousands of CDs and LPs. He put some music on while I was at his house. Most of the songs I hadn't heard before but the two songs I knew and liked were 'Where Have All the Cowboys Gone' by Paula Cole and The Verve's 'The Drugs Don't Work'.

I became good friends with Ray's family and went to see them every few weeks.

I made a decision to do my best to get my foot in door at Surf. I thought once I got in, it would be easy to prove what I can do in radio. However, not wanting to put all of my eggs in one basket, I thought it would be good to write to other radio stations and send them a tape of the programme I had made at New Wave.

Another thing I did was subscribe to *The Radio Magazine* and read it avidly every month. It contained news, features and job vacancies – and I felt part of the industry.

In making several more copies of my programme on tape I also got a booklet, from the Radio Authority, of all the commercial radio stations in the UK. What I didn't have was a CV.

This is where Stephen Holmes helped me a lot – one of the advertisers in the family newspaper, who offered a CV writing service. I phoned him up and explained my circumstances and he said he would be glad to help me. We ended up having a long conversation on the phone.

After we had chatted for over an hour, Stephen called me an inspiration. Being called inspirational made me feel a little odd because I thought, *what have I done? I haven't achieved anything yet.*

Stephen mentioned he was planning to come to meet my family and was looking forward to meeting me. The upshot of meeting Stephen was that we became friends and he didn't charge me for creating a really smart CV and covering letter. He said they were free of charge as long as I used them as a template to help others. I helped at least five people with their CVs and cover letters.

To make my CV and covering letter stand out I printed them on light blue paper. I sent my letter, CV and cassette tape to every radio station in London, as well as stations which were south-east of London. I also posted it to the managing director (MD) of Surf, who seemed to be operating from a residential address as they didn't have an office yet.

I was due to start working on the Spirit sports show on 6th September 1997 but the sports show was cancelled that week, due to the funeral of Lady Diana, Princess of Wales, so I started the next week.

It was great fun at Spirit the following Saturday. Kevin presented the sports show and Anthony, who was about my age, worked at Spirit during the week and helped out on the sports show as well. There were also two fifteen-year-oldgirls who gathered the local football scores, by phoning each club in the Sussex County League at half-time and full-time, which Anthony read out on air.

My task was to capture the Premiership audio reports from IRN. IRN provide news and sport for commercial radio stations and transmit audio via satellite. Therefore, to receive IRN audio, radio stations needed a satellite dish. You could then hear and record the audio feed through the studio desk.

IRN would have a reporter at each Premiership game. I sat in the production studio and recorded onto the playout system, each report IRN sent down the line. Then I told Kevin which game I had a new report for, that he could then play on air.

I had to ensure there wasn't a gap at the start or end of each report. Also I edited out any bad stumbles/mistakes the reporters made. It was pretty easy and I took to it like a duck to water.

The two studios at Spirit were equipped with Talkback (a button you press to talk to the person in the other studio. The studios had a window in between them and I sat adjacent to Kevin – I could then see if it was a good time to say something to him or whether he was about to do a link.

The way Audio Vault (the play-out system) worked, I had to create a virtual cart (file) for each game beforehand. I then had them all as a list and selected which cart to record onto as reports came down the line.

These were the Premiership fixtures on the day I started on the sports show: I don't recall if all ten games started at 3 o'clock but at least six of them did.

Leicester v Tottenham
Derby v Everton
C Palace v Chelsea
Coventry v Southampton
Barnsley v Aston Villa
Newcastle v Wimbledon
Man Utd v West Ham
Arsenal v Bolton
Liverpool v Sheffield Wednesday
Blackburn v Leeds

Before the show started I set up virtual carts and called them as follows:

S1 – Leicester v Tottenham
S2 – Derby v Everton
S3 – Crystal Palace v Chelsea
S4 – Coventry v Southampton
S5 – Barnsley v Aston Villa
S6 – Newcastle v Wimbledon

And so on...

Kevin and I also had a printed list of the fixtures, which included the name of the reporter at each game.

The only thing I found difficult the first week I did the sports show was my lack of football knowledge – and not knowing the ground name of each Premiership team.

When IRN fed a report down the line, the reporter would say an intro, along the lines of, "Hello network, it's Joe Bloggs at Filbert Street, with a report coming to you in three – two – one." It got me thinking, *where on earth is Filbert Street? Which game is it?*

Luckily, most of the reporters mentioned the team names of the game they were covering in their intro.

In case I missed the start of a report, I left a DAT tape continuously recording. If needed, I could then dub the report from the DAT tape onto the computer.

Still, on the second Saturday, I overcame my lack of football knowledge by including the ground name and the reporter, in the title of each cart. For example:

S1 – Leicester V Tottenham – Filbert Street – Joe Bloggs

Doing this solved the issue – and over time I learnt the ground names!

One of the most important things I had to do in helping out on the sports show was to ensure I spoke very clearly to Kevin. In letting him know which reports I had recorded, I would say something like, "There's another Chelsea goal on S-three. It's now three-nil."

Most of the reports ended with the reporter saying the score of the game – for example, "It's Crystal Palace nil, Chelsea three," – and this is what Kevin was expecting. However, sometimes a reporter would end by saying something other than the score. On these occasions, I had to tell Kevin what the last three or four words of the report were.

It wasn't unusual for IRN to feed a number of reports back to back, which could become a bit frantic. I had to really concentrate in recording the reports onto the correct carts. The more reports there were, the bigger the buzz I got. I loved working at Spirit and the teamwork it involved.

The sports show was between 2.00 pm and 6.00 pm on Saturday. During the last hour of the programme, we did a montage of three or four full-time Premiership reports. The montage was directly followed by the classified football results, which IRN used to do starting at exactly 5.30 pm. This was the sequence of events up to the montage and classified football results:

- Song
- Kevin's link into the ad break
- Ad break
- Jingle
- Montage of full-time reports (with music bed)
- Jingle
- IRN classified football results

As IRN started the classified football results at precisely 5.30 pm Kevin needed to know how long my montage was (it was always between two and three minutes). He could then work out what time he had to start the ad break.

Using Audio Vault allowed me to chain the reports together and the system would then display the total running time of the montage. As the reports were chained together, the system automatically played them back to back and I only had to press one button to start the first report.

The music bed we played underneath the reports came from a CD I cued up in my studio.

As I looked at the clock on the wall in front of me, Kevin told me when there were ten seconds remaining of the ad break – I started the bed at the same time that he started the jingle – then at the at the end of the jingle I fired the first report. It was as easy as that!

Due to the dreaded 'double press' syndrome, the first time I did the montage I made a slight mishap. Having not played anything on air before, my nerves were jangling and I had a trembling finger, waiting to press the button to start the bed. Instead of pressing the button once, I pressed it twice which started the bed (for the briefest of moments) and then stopped it!

Anthony was in the studio with me at the time and just started the bed again. Still, I beat myself up about it afterwards.

However, I did it fine the second week and didn't make the same mistake twice.

Me being me, it wasn't long before I asked Kevin to let me know the length of the ad break. This enabled me to do the back-timing and I told Kevin what time he needed to go into the ad break every week.

Working on the sports show required several skills; teamwork, good communication and technical skills, being organised and working well under pressure. Because I loved working in radio I was very good at it.

It makes me smile when I think what the deputy head at boarding school said to me, about not being organised enough to handle going to college!

I have always tended to be a perfectionist and I hate making mistakes in life. My perfectionism is most prevalent when working in radio because it requires pin-point accuracy.

The reason for my perfectionism is simple – I have never wanted anyone to think *Patrick can't help it, he's disabled.*

Over the last three years in property I have learnt that making a mistake is not a problem. It only becomes a problem when you don't learn from the mistake.

As Martin and Janet lived fairly close to Spirit I often went to see them after the sports show. The three of us went out in Brighton a couple of times. On one occasion we ended up going to the Gloucester nightclub. As I had never tried to dance before (without my crutches) I tried dancing with Janet. However, she couldn't support my weight and we both fell over laughing! I know the things I'm good at in life and dancing isn't one of them!

Martin and I also went out in Worthing a few times. I then started going out to pubs and clubs on my own.

Before getting into property investment – and learning about the law of attraction (the difference between pushing and pulling) – I spent so much time and energy – going out to pubs, looking for a girlfriend. Over several years I met so many drunk women who gave me their phone number, but who tended not to want to know me when I phoned them the next day. I got to know some women better than others – but I found the pain of being rejected is the worst pain in the world.

I didn't get much response from all of the letters I sent to at least twenty radio stations in 1997. Capital Radio in London wrote back to me saying they had put my tape (the programme I made at New Wave) forward for an award. I would have preferred it if Capital had written back offering me a job!

Nevertheless, it didn't deter me from arranging to visit a few stations. A station I went to twice was Talk Radio in London (catching the 6.30 am train from Shoreham). Talk Radio was fascinating. I sat in on Scott Chisholm's programme in the morning and then Tommy Boyd's show after lunch.

Each programme on the station used two studios. The presenter was in one studio, which had a few screens and a small console to put callers on the air. In the other studio were two people; a phone producer, who answered the calls and wrote a summary on the computer of each caller's point of view. The other person was known as a technical operator (TO), who sat in front of the main studio desk and 'drove it'.

I knew I could do the job of a TO. It didn't seem to be a very demanding role. All they appeared to do was start an ad break every fifteen minutes and play in the news bulletin every hour.

Both Scott Chisholm and Tommy Boyd were good and down to earth guys. Scott had a paper pad and made a note of every caller he spoke to. Tommy presented his shows standing up and was very humorous. Visually, Tommy reminded me of a scruffy bloke I knew in Shoreham.

The second time I went to Talk Radio, I knew that Ted was running an automated country music station from the same office – so I popped and said hello to him. I found it funny. Talk Radio had this big, modern and posh, open-plan office, which had quite a few people in it. Whilst Ted seemed to be tucked away and working on his own in what looked like a broom cupboard, with just him and three computers in it.

I was so determined to work in radio that I even drove to visit a tiny station in the middle of nowhere.

Towards the end of 1997 I had an appointment with Mr Patrick in Oswestry. He was pleased with how I was walking with my left foot and we discussed the possibility of further surgery. I was keen to have my hamstrings released/ lengthened but Mr Patrick said such an operation at my age was risky. He said the operation might cause more problems than it would solve.

He did mention the possibility of implanting some sort of bag into my stomach and injecting a muscle relaxant drug into it every few months. However, he said I would need to have such a high dosage of the drug, to have an effect on my muscles, that it would be too risky. It sounded really dangerous to me!

Therefore, I haven't had any more surgery on my feet or legs.

Mr Patrick did give me a pair of gaiters to stretch my hamstrings at night. He advised that a more passive stretch of eight hours was better than a thirty minute rigid stretch (which I got from the massive contraption that Peter built for me).

Gaiters are similar to leg splints but are made of material, which allowed my legs to bend slightly. In the back of each gaiter were three thin strips of metal and at the front were four Velcro straps.

Because the gaiters allowed my legs to bend a bit, it made the metal strips break through the material and dig into the back of my legs – which made my legs bleed. So we used pieces of foam to protect my legs.

My gaiters weren't the most comfortable of things but I got used to them and I wore them virtually every night (when I didn't go out somewhere) for three to four years. I preferred my gaiters to the massive contraption because I no longer had to spend an hour a day using it.

As I tended to sleep with my legs bent on the occasions when I didn't wear my gaiters it made my legs stiff the following day.

At first, Mum tried to put my gaiters on me but she didn't hold my right leg straight or do the gaiters up tight enough – which caused arguments. Therefore, Clare came through the back garden and put them on for me. She did each gaiter up really well – by putting her foot on my knee. Clare found it easy.

Unlike me, Clare has always been a bit of a stickler at time-keeping. We agreed she would come over at 10 o'clock every night but it was often 10.15 or later when I phoned her to say I was ready. But I really appreciated Clare putting on my gaiters.

Today, although I manage my hamstrings myself, they are still very stiff. With the advances in medicine and technology over the past sixteen years, I am interested to know about procedures which could loosen my hamstrings. Having straight knees would also make me a bit taller. At five foot one, I feel a bit short.

The operation on my foot in 1996 didn't reduce my energy consumption because I still use four times the amount of energy of an average person. The operation was a success in straightening my foot and eliminating the need for wearing a calliper. I can now wear a pair of normal shoes.

Although I don't drag my left foot anymore, I do walk on the inside of it slightly (the side of boot gets worn down). I wear steel toe capped boots because they are quite supportive and because I drag the front of my right boot up each step, when I walk up stairs.

The worst type of stairs are ones where each step has a lip on it because my right foot gets caught under each step. However, I have never come across stairs that I couldn't climb. It does take a lot of energy for me to climb stairs. I just see it as a few minutes of hard work.

Back in 1997, Clare gave birth to Oliver. It was nice having Clare living nearby and being around her kids when they were young. They were used to me speaking and walking differently to other people. The same is true about Martin and Janet's two kids and Ray's boys.

I remember playing 'the name game' with each of Clare's kids when they were about one and hadn't started talking yet. We would all be sat around and someone would say to Scott or Oliver (or Charlotte), "Where's Mummy?" and they looked at Clare, "Where's Daddy?" and they looked at Rupert, "Where's Grandma?" and they looked at Mum, or "Where's Patrick?" and they would look at me.

I felt there was something kind of magical about it. Albeit, only that they had a brain, intelligence and the ability to learn!

Once they were a bit older, they each asked Clare why I couldn't walk or talk properly. Clare simply explained what an umbilical cord is and that when I was born, it got caught around my neck and I couldn't breathe for a few minutes.

Elsewhere in 1997, in producing editorial content for the family newspaper John read a lot of the daily newspapers. Unbeknown to me, John had been building a folder of articles of people who had won compensation, following negligence at birth.

It prompted us to start to pursue a claim of negligence against the hospital where I was born. On the basis that they knew there was a problem, as Mum went to hospital with high blood pressure and they induced my birth – but there wasn't a doctor present at my birth who could have maybe got me breathing quicker than four minutes.

As I was on Income Support we got legal aid for a spiffy lawyer, who Mum and I went to visit in London Chambers. At which point, the lawyer had already retrieved some medical records and that's how I know about the circumstances of my birth. The lawyer also stated that I could win in excess of three quarters of a million pounds – but I think he just quoted that figure for the legal aid.

I don't know how someone can put a price on a person's life.

However, a couple of weeks later the lawyer said there wasn't enough evidence to pursue a case because Masons Hill Maternity Unit no longer existed!

It doesn't bother me. I know I can make £1 million myself.

Back at Spirit in December Kevin left the radio station. I was disappointed to see him leave because he was a good guy and we worked well together. During his last sports show Kevin mentioned to me that he was leaving the station. I appreciated him telling me because I don't think everyone at Spirit knew that he was going.

A few people covered the sports show until January when a new guy – called Andy Dancey – started as a presenter. Andy was a good, easy-going chap and we worked well together.

He seemed a bit unsure of me during his first show but once he saw me in action, he was at ease working with me.

When Andy started at Spirit he brought along a guy called Phil to help out on the sports show, who knew each other from doing hospital radio.

I don't remember talking to Phil much/at all at Spirit. He seemed like a quiet guy and he always wore a baseball cap. Until recently, I didn't even remember what it was that Phil did on the sports show – he read the local football scores.

Ironically years later, Phil and I became good friends when we did the sports show on another radio station. I think it's true to say that Phil is the person who knows me better than anyone else does. However after reading this book, *you* will also know me well!

A few weeks ago I saw Andy at Phil's fortieth birthday party. Andy now works on the technical side in television.

I recently asked Phil if we spoke to each other at Spirit. He said I once showed him how to record IRN reports onto the play-out system as I was going to be away one Saturday. It was rare for me to take a Saturday off from Spirit as I loved it so much, but I must have gone to see my Dad in France.

Dad split up with his girlfriend, Marie, sometime in 1998. I thought it was a shame because I found Marie to be a nice person.

Elsewhere in early 1998 Ray had had a few discussions with the MD of Surf and it was looking positive for Ray becoming the station/sales manager. Ray also mentioned to me that the MD was going to contact me, after Ray had told him about my ability and enthusiasm to work in radio.

The internet was in its infancy and the family business enlisted an American guy called Carl who lived in America, to set up a website for the business/newspaper. As John's brother (Norman) was interested and had some knowledge of the internet he also became involved with the website.

Over at Liz and John's house one morning, after Liz had got up, Nan was nowhere to be found. Worried, and not knowing what to do, or where on earth Nan was, Liz phoned Shoreham police station. The Police said they had found her wandering around in the street in the early hours of the morning in her nightie. As Nan was confused, didn't know her name or where she lived, all the police could do was to take her to the police station.

We had resisted putting Nan in a home for years. However, after getting up in the night and letting herself out of the house, it was obvious the time had come to do so. It was emotionally difficult but once we found a nice home in Shoreham for her, there was also a sense of relief that we no longer had the stress of looking after her.

The staff at the care home were really good but I found going to visit Nan distressing (which made me feel sick). It was a Victorian house which always stank of toilet air freshener, there were pots of potpourri everywhere and the place had flowery furniture and curtains. Not my type of décor, I'm a more modern guy!

There were five or six residents, all with Alzheimer's. It was a depressing place because they just seemed to be sitting around waiting to die. The staff were not bad, they often talked to the residents and made them laugh, and let them out into the garden. But there's not much you can do with old people who have lost their mind. Nevertheless, I went to visit Nan every week or two.

By February Surf had contacted Ray to say they had decided to appoint somebody else as station/sales manager. It was very disappointing (for Ray and for me).

It was, therefore, a surprise, in early March, when I received a phone call from Vic, the MD of Surf, inviting me to go and meet him at home. I arranged to visit him a few days later.

I felt very anxious for the next few days, leading up to meeting Vic. He lived in a ground floor apartment off Brighton seafront. I remember nervously walking up the few steps to his front door and ringing the bell.

When Vic answered the door he was surprised to see me. He said he wasn't feeling very well and had forgotten about our meeting. He asked me if I would mind waiting outside for a few minutes whilst he put some other clothes on.

When Vic let me in, I was only there for about five minutes. He said the station was going to be launching towards the end of the month and they needed someone (eg me) to record a lot of music onto the play-out system, as all of the songs were going to be played from the computer. Vic said he would get one of the on-air programming team to give me a call nearer the time.

Vic said they would pay me £3 an hour to record the music. I thought, *that's below the minimum wage.* However, I was so eager to get into the station and prove what I could do, I didn't think to ask Vic for more money.

I began to worry after a week because I hadn't heard from anyone at Surf. *If they're launching the station by the end of the month*, I thought, *why haven't they got me in to record music onto the system yet?* I remember meeting Ray one lunchtime in mid-March in McDonald's at Brighton Marina (as Ray was working for a Brighton Magazine).

My confidence was extremely low, I felt sick and my nervous cough was really bad.

Me: "They're not going to call me, are they?

Ray: "Just be patient."

A few days later I had a call from Jason asking when I could come into the station. My foot was in the door at Surf and I was feeling very confident!

Patrick Souiljaert

Chapter 9

Disclaimer: I worked at Surf (predominantly as a volunteer) for two and a half years until September 2000. It was my choice to work at Surf for as long as I did and I could have left the station at any time. I bear no ill will towards any of the people I worked with. The radio station was sold a few months after I left the company. I have had no affiliations or dealings with the station or any subsequent management personnel since I left in September 2000.

The premises of Surf were located in the centre of Brighton, where there was no off-road parking. I therefore parked my car in a side street, about twenty yards away from the radio station. Once inside the building, there were five steps up to a long corridor, leading into a big, wooden floored, open-plan office. At the front of the office was a sofa and the reception desk. To the right were a group of desks for the salespeople.

Further in, on the right, were three little enclosed offices, for the station/sales manager, MD and finance guy respectively. On the left were a set of desks for the programming team/presenters and the news team. Heading forward was a small kitchen area leading to the carpeted stairs, which were at the back of the building. The studios were upstairs.

The distance from my car to the stairs must have been about fifty yards, which I found pretty tiring to walk.

The first time I went into the station I was greeted by Jason, who was one of the presenters. Upon reaching the bottom of the stairs, Jason asked, "Are you going to be alright going up the stairs? There's quite a lot of them."

I looked up through the centre of the stairs. *Wow, that's a long way up!* I thought. However, I replied, "Yes, I'll be fine. I can get to anywhere I want to go in life."

There were five flights of stairs, each containing five or six steps. Each flight was at 90 degrees to the previous one, meaning the stairs went up in a square formation.

The stairs had a wooden hand rail, held up by a series of white metal posts. I walked up the stairs by putting my right arm on the hand rail and holding a metal post, as I walked up the stairs – and holding both of my crutches in my left hand.

I was feeling so confident and eager to see the studios that I sprinted up the five flights of stairs.

Upstairs was a toilet, four studios and a small office. However, Surf only used two studios. The other two studios and the office were used by a separate production company.

I was surprised when I walked into the studios because the studio desk in both of them was quite high. They had been built for people to use standing up. However, there was a wooden stool which I managed to heave myself onto to sit in front of the desk.

Jason said there were already quite a few songs on the play-out system but there were a lot more that needed to be recorded onto it.

After we chatted about radio for a bit, Jason briefly showed me how ENCO DAD (the play-out system) worked. Having never used a touch-screen system before I thought it was magic!

I took to ENCO DAD like a duck to water. It wasn't long before I knew it like the back of my hand. It was so straightforward.

My first impression of the station was that it was a friendly and relaxed place to work.

I began working at Surf a week before the station launched. For the first couple of days I was recording songs onto the play-out system in the on-air studio (studio 1) but after that I always worked from the production studio (studio 2).

Both studios had essentially the same equipment in them; two CD players and two vinyl turntables. The ENCO DAD monitor sat on top of the pod which housed the CD players.

Everything about the station looked cheap. For example, there was no talkback facility between the two studios, the air conditioning units in them were noisy (not ideal for presenters doing links on the radio or someone reading the news!). Also the desks and chairs in the office downstairs looked cheap.

Over the first week I recorded numerous songs from CD onto ENCO DAD. At the time, I described it as playing my favourite computer game while listening to great music all day.

For each song I recorded I needed to set a couple of markers, which was easy using the touch-screen. The first marker was the intro time – the point in the song where the vocals start. This gave presenters a countdown of how long they could talk for over the beginning of the song.

The second marker – called the segueway point – was used when the system was playing songs in automation. The segueway marker went near the end of the song – and was the point at which the next item in the log (commonly a jingle or song) started to play.

For each song, I wrote down:
- The cut number I recorded the song onto (every piece of audio on the play-out system had a unique number)
- The length of the song
- The length of the intro time
- How the song ended (whether it had a slow fade or an ended with a beat)

When I started at Surf I felt really happy and confident. I felt I had achieved something monumental – something someone in my position wouldn't normally achieve. Now that I was in radio, I set myself another goal. I wanted to show people what I could do. I wanted to gain responsibility for playing out a show on the radio (similar to the show I saw Gary doing at Southern FM). I knew I could do it – my goal was to prove it.

The day the radio station launched was memorable. I felt part of the station. People knew I was very good in the studio and it seemed that I was well respected. Someone actually said that the radio station could not have launched if I hadn't recorded so many songs onto the system.

It was funny after the station started because I still had a lot of songs to record but people kept coming into the production studio, needing to use it. Surf had a twenty-five minute magazine show called *The List*, every weekday evening. There were often times during the day when people who worked on the programme and the news team both wanted to use the production studio. It became like a battle!

They reached an agreement whereby *The List* team could use the studio for the first forty minutes of every hour and news had it for the last twenty minutes,

The only thing I found difficult about working in the studio was having to get onto the high stool. Hence, I went out and bought a little desk and an office chair, which someone took up to studio 2 for me.

It worked and I overcame the problem of nearly falling over each time I got onto the stool. The desk I bought was small enough for it not to be in the way. It was at a right angle to, and at the end of the studio desk, facing the window into studio 1.

When I was in the studio, someone lifted the ENCO DAD screen down onto my little desk, which also had a pull-out draw for the computer keyboard. I sat in my chair, with my feet on the floor, I was well balanced. When I wasn't in the studio people put the computer screen back up onto the pod.

I built a good relationship with people at Surf. It seemed like the station relied heavily on volunteers. I think people saw Surf as a stepping stone to progress in radio.

Often when someone came to do something in the production studio, I offered to do it for them. As they always had other things to do and knowing that I was very competent, they were happy for me to help them.

I spent my time editing interviews, recording news cuts, which IRN fed every hour, sat in on interviews which were pre-recorded for *The List* and helped the news guys record bulletins. Around it all, I recorded more songs onto the system. I was loving it.

In the week during the station launch, Surf held a couple of launch parties at a nightclub. On one of the evenings, while I was sitting on the edge of the dancefloor, this girl came up to me. She was signing at me, as if I were deaf. The only sign language I know is of the one and two-fingered variety!

I said to her that I wasn't deaf. As the music was very loud we went outside for a chat. Somehow, we ended up seeing each other! I couldn't believe my luck, it happened so naturally. Her name was Hannah and she worked with deaf people. She mentioned she had recently split up with her boyfriend.

I had recently bought my first mobile phone. Hannah would phone me up and say, "I'm meeting some friends for a drink, do you want to join us?" so I did. I would go and meet them and then Hannah and I would end up alone, kissing and cuddling each other. It felt SO nice. We saw each other two or three times a week.

Life was good. I sort of had a girlfriend and I loved working in radio. Something that I hadn't experienced before happened (I didn't know what it was at the time) – I started to live in the present moment. I wasn't worried about anything anymore. No longer did I feel sick or throw up. My insomnia had disappeared and I had loads of energy. I was happy to let my relationship with Hannah develop naturally.

I remember sitting with Hannah in a Brighton pub one Saturday evening when we got chatting to a woman, who was sitting nearby. After a few minutes:

Woman: "You two look really good together."

Hannah: "Thank you, Patrick's my boyfriend and we're very happy."

As we then kissed each other.

I don't need to worry about finding a girlfriend anymore, I thought. *I can just relax now.* I remember telling Ray about Hannah.

When I started at Surf I worked for thirty-two days in a row – often for twelve hours a day. I was in the zone and loving it. Someone in the office went out and did a sandwich 'lunch run' every day. The song "No Way" by Freak Power was on heavy rotation and it became like an anthem in the office. It was a really good atmosphere.

People got used to me walking up stairs every morning. They saw that I was independent, really good in the studio and that I didn't need any help – hence they just left me to do what I did.

Once I got up the stairs in the morning I stayed upstairs all day. Being left handed, with the rail on the left, made walking down the stairs easier than climbing them.

For the first couple of weeks Surf mainly played indie music (which I was really into). However, it then became a more dance-orientated station and played more chart songs during the day. After seven o'clock there were a number of nightclub DJs who each did a show one evening a week.

The nightclub DJs brought their own records in, as their shows weren't playlisted and they could play what they wished. Although the evening DJs didn't play songs from ENCO DAD, they needed to use the system for adverts and jingles.

However, it seemed none of the DJs had been shown how to use ENCO DAD or the studio desk. Therefore, being my helpful self, I taught them – and they respected me.

Like many commercial radio stations, in their licence application Surf had a commitment to broadcast hourly news bulletins between certain hours. After 7.00 pm Surf broadcast the news bulletins that IRN provided, starting precisely on the hour. I showed the evening DJs how to bring up the IRN news, where the news jingle was, how to back-time and the like.

On Saturdays I was at Surf in the morning and drove to Chichester at lunchtime for the sports show at Spirit in the afternoon. I felt awesome working at two radio stations. One Saturday morning, Alison Hulme came into Surf for a voice test to read the news. However, she didn't end up working for the station. I was the only person from New Wave who was working at Surf.

After doing the sports show at Spirit one Saturday I went to see Martin and Janet. Whenever I went to see them I always liked playing hide and seek with Ben and making him laugh. I mentioned to Janet that I was thinking about finding a flat to rent in Brighton or Hove. I was on Income Support and was eligible for housing benefit. Janet said she liked house hunting and offered to come and help me look with Ben.

I was quite naive and hadn't thought about, or looked into, it before Janet and Ben came to Shoreham and we went to a few letting agents in Hove. What we found was that there weren't a lot of ground floor flats in Brighton and Hove, with off-road parking.

And obviously, it wasn't simply a case of walking into letting agents and asking "Have you got any suitable flats? Can we go and view them now?" I think we saw one grotty flat that day. We mainly went into letting agents. Still, it was nice spending the day with Janet and Ben.

Moving out of home was just an idea I had at that stage. It's not something I had considered carefully. Not having a proper job, I wasn't earning any/much money.

The day I went flat hunting (with Janet and Ben) must have been the first day I took off from Surf, after having worked thirty-two days in a row. Throughout the day I received three phone calls from people at Surf, who were trying to do things that I normally did, asking me how to do them! It made me feel valued at the station.

Things started to go downhill after about six weeks at the station, when I had a meeting with Frank, the station/sales manager, to discuss how much they were going to pay me for recording music onto ENCO DAD. I found it odd that the meeting was with Frank and not Vic (the MD). Vic was the person had offered me the job and the only dealing I had had with Frank was saying hello to him in passing. Frank never seemed to have much input on the programming side of the station

The meeting didn't go terribly well. First, we had a dispute over how many songs I had recorded onto the system. Jason sat in on the meeting and I was astonished when he sided with Frank, arguing that I hadn't recorded as many songs as I was claiming. I said to them, "I can go upstairs, look on ENCO DAD and prove how many songs I have recorded..."

However, Frank was only willing to pay me £200. When I mentioned I had been working for twelve hours a day and that I had been doing so many things in the studio for other people – and I had more songs to record, Frank replied, "We only offered to pay you to record music onto the system. All of the other things you've done, you've done voluntarily. Other people are paid to do their jobs here. And we can't pay you to record any more songs."

it seemed to me they knew I was eager and that I would work for free.

The thing that really hurt was when Frank said, "Thank you very much for everything you've done here. We would like you to come in for one day a week from now on."

Can you imagine how worthless I felt?

For a brief moment I thought about walking out of the station there and then. But I would have felt a failure had I done so. Also, I was absolutely determined to achieve my goal and prove what I could do.

I didn't consider that Frank was my boss so I just carried on going into Surf every day. However, the meeting with Frank began to poison my mind again; I felt unvalued and like I had done something wrong. I started beating myself up, feeling sick and vomiting again. My confidence had disappeared.

I remember meeting up with Hannah one evening. The meeting with Frank was still on my mind, it was making me feel sick and I looked ill. Hannah asked, "What's wrong?"

It was weird. I knew I wasn't happy with the way Surf were treating me but I didn't know what was making me feel sick. My thoughts of being useless, worthless and that I had done something wrong were so subconscious. I felt really weak.

I didn't know what to say to Hannah so I replied, "I'm alright, I'm just not happy at Surf anymore.' I wish I had told her about the meeting with Frank. Hannah and I may have met up one more time after that but then I never heard from her again.

It was very bizarre. Having given her a lift home on various occasions I knew where Hannah lived and I had her home phone number. I called her several times but there was no answer so I went to her house. I think it was a neighbour of hers who said that Hannah had moved out.

Who knows what happened to her. Was she on the rebound from breaking up with her boyfriend and did she go back to him? I don't know.

It really hurt me and I blamed myself for messing things up with Hannah. My mindset plummeted even further. After seeing each other for about a month I thought, *at least I know what happiness is now. I've just got to find it again.*

Although I kept going into Surf, over the remaining two plus years I became more and more demoralised. It was grinding me down and I gradually spent fewer hours there. In the end I was only going in for one afternoon per week.

I did get on with a lot of people there. Working with the news guys was good fun. They did an extended five minute bulletin which I helped to pre-record. The bulletin was in a number of segments, each having a separate bed. I started and played all of the news clips in the bulletin for them – and then edited the whole thing together.

On one occasion, Gavin had a story which made me burst out laughing every time he attempted to read it. In the end I went out of the studio while he read it. The story was about a drunk guy who fell off the roof of his house, after he climbed onto it and attempted to fix his television aerial. The mental image it paints in my mind still makes me smile!

I often helped another newscaster with a live two minute bulletin at 7.00 pm.

Other people I got on well with at the station were:

Joanna – the breakfast show presenter, who had a 'name that song in one beat' feature. I found a good snippet of songs and saved them onto a separate cut on ENCO DAD for her to use. The funny thing was, Joanna often left for the day shortly after 10.00 am. Once I started going into the station a bit later. I hardly saw Joanna – but I was still finding songs for her to use.

Karen – who managed most of the volunteers. I remember chatting to her in the kitchen area downstairs, when she asked me, "What's your background?"

I glanced behind me then looked back at her and said, "A white wall and an untidy office!"

Carly – a volunteer for about six months before she got a job in London. Carly was a really nice and intelligent girl. We got on very well and were the same age. She called me Paddy, which is not a name I like but I didn't mind Carly calling me that!

Carly hosted a leaving party dinner when she got her job in London and invited a few people. Never being a fussy eater, I'll eat just about everything. However, the one thing I don't like is curry due to the smell it produces (I do like naan bread though). Curry is what Carly had made for that evening! I didn't know what to do! Not wanting to offend her I ate it. It was quite a mild curry and I said it was very nice!

I did some stuff with Mick Fuller, one of the freelance dance DJs who also owned a record shop. Mick compiled a weekly top 20 dance chart, which somebody else presented on Sundays. I helped Mick record the new releases onto ENCO DAD and then created the playlist/log, containing the twenty songs. Mick also provided a laugh every week!

Darren was a good guy. He presented *The List* and often pre-recorded interviews in the afternoon, which I sat in on. Beverly Knight, who was nice and bubbly, came in two or three times promoting her latest singles

The funniest person I met was comedian Jerry Sadowitz, After Darren had done a good interview with him, Jerry was even funnier afterwards. He had Darren and I in tears of laughter with his sharp gags!

An odd bloke was Uri Geller. He came into the studio saying he had called the police because he found a ladies handbag walking into the station! He then picked up a teaspoon, out of a cup on the windowsill and bent it. That was nothing. I was bending tablespoons when I was five-years-old!

The band that I walked straight past in my first week at the station was the Stereophonics. Kelly Jones said "Alright mate?" to me, as I walked past them which I acknowledged with a smile. I didn't who they were at the time. Years later I saw them in concert at The Brighton Centre.

I was still doing a lot of things and helping people in the studio but it was making me feel sick. Subconsciously, I was thinking, *I'm just helping people do their job.* Some people at Surf thought I was a bit weird because it wasn't uncommon for me to have a sick look on my face.

Among the volunteers at the radio station were two guys; Seth, who I knew from New Wave, and who joined Surf a few months after I did. The other chap was called Kevin who, like me, did technical/production work. Unlike me, they could run up and down the stairs all day long. It made me feel that they were better than me and that I had to compete with them.

On Friday evenings a group of people from the station went to the pub. I didn't really like some of the people who normally went but I thought it was better than sitting at home.

On one occasion, I was asked if I were gay and they recommended that I tried having gay sex. I thought it was an odd thing to ask me because they knew I had been seeing Hannah. I replied that I wasn't gay and had no interest in having gay sex. I don't think any homophobic people would have lasted very long working at Surf.

Up until 2000, when I had some counselling (to help me stop vomiting), and I consequently learnt why some gay men find me attractive, I thought it odd that men often tried to chat me up.

Sometimes the pub would lead onto a nightclub, which I went to a few times. I avoided going to gay nightclubs because I thought, *I'll be like honey to bees*. However, it wasn't uncommon for me to get approached by gay men in any nightclub, trying to chat me up. It was unnerving because I didn't understand why I was attracting gay men.

On one occasion I was sitting on my own in a Brighton nightclub when a bloke came to sit next to me:

Gay man: "So how long have you known that you're gay?"

Me: (calmly and with authority) "I am not gay."

Never have I seen someone move away from me as fast as he did!

It prompted me to start going out to nightclubs in Worthing, *thinking I met Hannah in a nightclub, so I can probably meet another girl in one.* I found the nightclub opposite Worthing train station was good. Having been to it before with Martin, I could park my car nearby and the club had two dancefloors.

One time at that club I bumped into a girl who said, "Hello Patrick Sue-lee-art, how the devil are you?" I looked at her blankly:

Me: "Who are you?"

Claire: "I'm Claire, Ricky's sister."

(I met Claire when I went to Ricky's twelfth birthday party, when I was at secondary school.)

Me: "How do you remember how to say my surname?"

Claire: "I'll never forget your name!"

We chatted for a few minutes. Claire said that Ricky was a white van driver and that she managed a hair salon.

It's not uncommon for me to bump into people who know me but who I sometimes struggle to recognise! In trying to identify them, I'll ask a leading question like, "What have you been up to lately?" It sometimes works!

One Friday evening, people from Surf went to a pub which was on a pedestrian precinct. I parked my car in front of, what appeared to be, a narrow pedestrian alleyway, a short distance from the pub.

On leaving the pub past eleven o'clock, we all went our separate ways. As I was walking back to my car I did a double-take because my car was no longer there! *Where's my car gone?* I thought. *What do I do? What do I do?*

I phoned Brighton Police Station and said, "Please can you help me. I have Cerebral Palsy, I walk with crutches and cannot walk very far. My car has been stolen or towed away. I need some help." And I told them where I was.

The lady I spoke to said, "Don't worry, stay where you are and someone will be along to help you in a few minutes."

Picture this scene – it's about 11.30 pm on a Friday night in the centre of Brighton – and there are lots of people around. A police van pulls up, two police officers get out the front of it. They come over to speak to me and then hold me under both of my arms and help into the back of the police van! I found it hilarious.

At the station the police ascertained that my car had been towed away. I phoned Clare: "Hi, I'm sorry to call you so late. Don't worry, I'm fine but I'm at Brighton Police Station... My car has been towed away. Please could you come and pick me up and give me a lift to the pound..."

At least the pound was on the way home. I made an expensive mistake – it cost me over a hundred quid to get my car back. The people at the pound said they had to remove my car because it was blocking someone's driveway. I had seen it – it looked like a long and narrow alleyway. It didn't look wide enough to fit a car down.

In my defence, I have got a depth-perception issue, probably due to my lazy left eye. I went to an optician in my mid-twenties, who said that I should have worn a patch over my right eye when I was a kid (to make my left eye get out of bed).

Back at the station – the radio station, not the police station – I started taking in my own sandwiches because the daily lunch run didn't last long. Also, it became apparent that I was unable to rely on anyone to make a coffee. Hence, I bought a flask and made coffee in it every day, before walking up the stairs, carrying my flask and sandwiches in my rucksack.

A couple of months after my meeting with Frank, the ENCO DAD monitor in the production studio developed a loose connection – it had a blue-green appearance and would obviously need to be repaired.

Soon after I arrived at the station one morning, Jason informed me, "Vic wants to see you in his office."

When I went into his office, Vic made it perfectly clear that I was a volunteer at the station and that I was free to leave the premises at any time. He went on to say, if I wanted to stay that the ENCO DAD screen was not to be moved under any circumstances.

Writing about it now, I wouldn't put myself through the same again and part of me thinks I should have walked out there and then. However, I think I would have felt like a failure, had I done so, because I had set myself a goal – and I was determined to achieve it.

I have to find a solution, I thought. Therefore, I phoned the ENCO DAD supplier and got the cost of another touchscreen monitor and a switchbox. I then contacted Scope (the charity for people with CP) and they agreed to pay for the new equipment.

Then I went to see Vic to ask him if Surf would lend me the money, while it came through from Scope, so that I didn't have to work standing up. Vic said no.

I think the mistake I made was not asking Vic for more money, when I first met him. I just accepted him offering me £3 an hour to record songs onto the system. In not asking for more money, Vic realised that he could 'walk all over me'.

For six weeks, I used the touch-screen monitor standing up. I alternated every few minutes between working standing up and having a rest sitting down.

When the money came through from Scope, the ENCO DAD supplier said, "We haven't got a new fourteen inch (or it may have been fifteen inch) monitor in stock at the moment – but we're got a reconditioned seventeen inch one you can have for the same price."

Therefore, in the production studio there were two ENCO DAD screens – the 17 inch monitor on my little desk and the smaller one up on the pod and a switch box to switch between the two.

The thing that really annoyed me about Vic was he knew that I was intelligent. Several times, throughout the two and a half years I was there, Vic said to me "Find yourself a niche and I'll pay you." At the time, it made me think *what am I meant to do when there are five flights of stairs?*

Life at home was no picnic either. Mum had come home from the office one day in 1998, in a rage and said to me, "I've had a major argument with Liz and John, but I don't want it to affect you."

She then went into the kitchen, slamming the door closed. *Oh Christ*, I thought, *what's happened now?*

It took her under five minutes to come and have a rant at me and said: "I needed to send an urgent email but Damian was playing a game on the computer. So I asked him to get off the computer so I could send my email, at which point John shouted at me across the whole office, "Don't you speak to my son like that."

She went on raging: "So I stormed out of the office, kicking the bin over on my way out."

After pausing momentarily for breath: "How dare John talk to me like that? How fucking dare he? And why didn't Liz – my own sister – why didn't Liz walk out of the office with me?"

This will probably blow over in a few days, I thought. But it didn't. It never has been resolved – or forgotten.

In the days following the antagonistic event in the office, Mum constantly made out that John was the most evil person on earth, proclaiming her innocence, and what a terrible injustice had been visited on her – and how disgusted she was with Liz for not coming to see her to apologise for not supporting her.

When Liz did come over to see Mum, about a week after the altercation in the office, carrying a plant as a gift, the pair of them stood at the front door talking for a few minutes, but Mum didn't accept Liz's apology or the plant.

Mum told me that Liz hadn't come over soon enough to apologise and that it wasn't sincere enough. What Mum wanted was for Liz to take her side in the dispute.

A week or so later, Mum received a softly worded letter from John, who apologised and included some family photos of Liz, John and Mum together. In his letter John wrote something along the lines of, 'You should admit you are partly at fault.' Mum said to me if John hadn't said that, she would have forgiven him.

I continued to socialise with my cousins and to have dinner at Liz and John's house with them all on Sunday evenings. However, within a few weeks Sunday dinner became uncomfortable when Mum was being discussed and badmouthed around the table. Therefore, I stopped having dinner at their house. Soon after that, tensions started to build up with my cousins and so I also stopped socialising with them.

Clare and Becky, who had always got on well, started to distance themselves from each other.

Mum started to work from home to fulfil her obligations in publishing a newspaper every two weeks. She lost contact with Liz (living two houses from one another). It was the start of formal and hostile letters being delivered between John and Mum.

What a way to run a business – which lumbered on for a couple of years.

What had always been a very close family (especially Mum, Liz and John) was now a divided one.

It was a horrible situation to be caught in. It was obvious to Clare and I that Mum was being closed-minded, not accepting any responsibility, but we both felt some loyalty towards her. Mum dragged Clare and I down with her – especially me because we were living together.

Mum became consumed with the belief that John and Liz were 100% to blame and that she was faultless. It became her life – trying to convince other people that she was the victim of a great injustice.

Liz and Mum used to regularly speak to Great Aunt Doris on the phone. After a while Doris got fed up of listening to Mum going on and on about the situation – so Doris decided to sever ties with her.

The situation didn't help Mum's feelings towards Rupert. Whenever anything bad was said about Rupert, Clare would leap to his defence. It created more tension between Clare and Mum.

Over the weeks, months and years, Mum broke the relationships she had with her family and virtually all of the friends she had at the time.

The only person Mum had left was me – and living together became even more strained. I felt sorry for her because I thought, *all she's got to do is see sense.* I spent twelve years trying to help her.

Even after I moved out, Mum still used me as a metaphorical doormat, to wipe her feet on and as her emotional punch-bag. She would not leave me alone.

It was the worst twelve years of my life. I kept trying to get her to see that life isn't so black and white and trying to get her to take some responsibility. However, she wouldn't take on board anything I said. Instead she said I wasn't trying hard enough in my life.

I got caught in another vicious circle. I kept thinking, *why isn't anything I do or say helping her? I'm not trying hard enough. I need to try harder to help her.* My mindset was getting more and more infected.

In late 2010, I got myself out of the vicious circle I was in with Mum. Rarely did I vomit in public, but Mum had made me so stressed that I was unable to contain myself. I went out for a meal, three days after my birthday, when I vomited at the table, in front of my friends and the other people in the restaurant. It was probably as embarrassing as the time I peed myself in my classroom when I was ten years old.

It was the final straw. I had to take defining action.

I emailed Mum, told her what happened in the restaurant and I wrote: "From this moment on, I have taken away your right to contact me. I am forbidding you from contacting me again. I will contact you when I'm ready to do so."

After sending that email I knew I had probably gotten through to Mum because she didn't reply to my email.

Then a couple of days later, I suddenly realised I was feeling relaxed and that I hadn't thrown up in the last two days. For sixteen years, having never worked out the reason why I kept vomiting, I realised, due to her negativity and making me feel bad about myself, Mum was largely the cause of it.

Mum caused me so much pain and stress for so many years. When I freed myself from her, I stopped vomiting overnight.

What I find interesting is, by getting into property investment I have learnt so much about people and human behaviour. Over the last four years I have changed so much, and writing this book has also helped me to become at peace with myself.

I have no anger towards Mum because I have overcome everything – and because what's done is done (the past cannot be changed).

I love my mum and my wish for her is that she becomes at peace with herself and with her sister and brother-in-law. Liz and John are now approaching their mid seventies and are both in poor health. I urge Mum to forgive and forget the past and to make peace with my aunt and uncle. I also urge Liz and John to embrace Mum. The only time that truly matters in life is RIGHT NOW.

Back in the late nineties, to add to the family/business complexity, a dispute emerged between Carl and Norman (the American guy hired to set up the website, and John's brother). It ended up with Carl taking the family business to court over the ownership of a website domain name (and possibly the website content)!

To the best of my knowledge, all Carl wanted was the domain name. In my opinion, it should have never gone to court. It seemed liked Norman had only been brought into the website build because he was interested in the Internet and had limited knowledge of it. I don't know what he contributed.

Throughout the proceedings Mum and Carl remained good friends (at the same time and as he was suing her business)! She liked having an ally.

Then, another dispute started between John (the family business) and Norman! I don't know if this dispute went anywhere – or if John and Norman are on speaking terms today.

My family is more dysfunctional than *The Simpsons*!

Back in radio-land, I was still doing the sports show at Spirit until the day someone at the station, for some reason, decided to get rid of all the volunteers who helped with the show. It was disappointing because I really enjoyed it. I must have helped out on the sports show for about a year or more.

Still, at Surf I was now playing-out a show on Sunday afternoons. Chris Philips, a presenter on Kiss 100 in London, came into Surf one evening every week to pre-record a two hour show. He recorded the show in six segments to cater for three ad breaks per hour.

I suggested to Chris that he record a separate dry link, which I could play over the last song of the show – and backtime it into the ad break, before the IRN news bulletin. Chris was a good guy and he respected me. He always gave me a mention, calling me his producer, in that last link.

I played-out Chris's show on Sunday afternoon for quite a few months. In, doing so, it could be said that I had achieved the goal I had set myself. Not so.

Doing Chris's show was kind of like the job the technical operator did at Talk Radio. It only required pressing a couple of buttons every fifteen minutes or so – one button to start an ad break and one to start the next segment of the show (and working out a bit of back-timing). It was a pretty boring job.

In my mind it was very clear what my goal was. I wanted to regularly drive a show, along the lines of the one I did at New Wave – whereby someone else just pre-recorded dry links and played-out the show. However, it was going to be easier to do on Surf because everything was on computer.

Whenever I played-out a live show I always did it from the production studio (so that I could sit on my chair, using my ENCO DAD monitor). Switching the production studio into the live one (and vice versa) just entailed pressing a button in both studios (and having a fader open during the switchover). Easy stuff!

About eighteen months into my time at Surf, Frank left the station and a new station/sales manager arrived. I got on with the new guy (Jeff) better than I did with Vic and Frank.

At some point, Surf started paying me the grand sum of £15 per week. The work involved dubbing two shows from DAT tape onto ENCO DAD – and playing a Surf jingle every ten to fifteen minutes.

One of the shows was two hours long, the other was just an hour. Both shows were in segments, which I had to create a log for, and insert the adverts. It was pretty boring, especially since I wasn't into weird dance music (mainly drum and bass style).

Throughout the two and a half years at Surf I applied for various studio production jobs. When I went to one interview in London I discovered they wanted more of a radio engineer. It wasn't so much being able to work in radio studios, it was a case of being able to build them!

I had an interview at Virgin Radio when Chris Evans was the breakfast show presenter. It was at the time when the breakfast show was being simultaneously broadcast on Sky One TV. The interview was for someone to play the ad breaks on Sky One – ensuring that they were the same length as the ad breaks on the radio. Needless to say, I didn't get the job but I could have done it easily. Another interview was at Classic FM, where there were nice studios.

The place I really wanted to get into was the BBC. With it being big and an equal opportunities company, I thought I would have good prospects there.

Over a period of weeks and months, I built up a good rapport, speaking on the phone to a guy who was quite senior (or I thought he was quite senior) in the BBC's HR department.

When I came to apply to go on a twelve week course to become a studio producer with the BBC, I was meticulous in completing the application form, which Damian helped me with. Before submitting it, I sent it to my contact in the HR department, who said my application form looked great. However, I never even got an interview.

The best radio job interview I had was in 1999 or 2000, at BBC Radio Oxford. The job was for a studio assistant, on £11,000 per year.

When I got some way up the M40 motorway, driving to Oxford I tuned into the radio station, to get the feel of it. It was predominately speech based with a bit of music. I heard them play 'My Heart Will Go On' by Celine Dion (I'm not her biggest fan!).

I was feeling confident and the interview started well. There were three people interviewing me:

Interviewer: "Where do you work?"

Me: "I work at Surf in Brighton."

Interviewer: "Surf... isn't that a washing powder?"

It made me laugh!

After asking me a few more questions, it was time to drive a mock news bulletin, which one of the interviewers read.

I sat at the studio desk, opposite the guy reading the news. There were three news stories, each having a piece of audio to go with it. I had a paper copy of the news script so that I knew when to play each clip. All I had to do was to play the clips and close and open the guy's microphone during each clip.

Before starting the bulletin (which they got me to record on reel-to-reel tape), they spent two or three minutes showing me the computer play-out system, and how to load up and unload the news clips. I found it easy. *Why are they spending so long showing me this?* I thought.

Then they asked me, "Do you understand how to load and unload the clips?" I thought, *they're going to get me to do something!* I had the three clips loaded up and we started the bulletin.

When I played the first news clip and had the microphone closed, the guy said to me, "I'm going to drop the second story and just do the third one, is that okay?' It was a piece of cake!

After the bulletin, they gave me about half an hour to write a thirty second promo and asked me to state any music or sound effects I would have with it. The trailer was to promote an up and coming royal anniversary event that they were going to do a programme on. Not being much of a royalist didn't stop me coming up with something that I was pleased with.

Then they asked me a few more questions. One of which was:

Interviewer: "If you were producing a show on the station, can you give me an example of a song you would include?"

Me: (with no hesitation!) "Celine Dion – My Heart Will Go On."

I was very pleased with how the interview had gone and therefore a bit gutted when I didn't get the job.

However, I managed to get feedback from one of the guys who had interviewed me. He said they were extremely impressed with me and the person who got the job just had a bit more experience. He went on to say that thirty people had applied for the job, ten were interviewed and I was in the shortlist of three people.

Another place I drove to was Television Centre in London. I went for an interview, working on the BBC News website. It was for a role writing the headlines which appear near the top of the BBC News homepage (which often includes 'BREAKING NEWS' in red and white).

There were three people interviewing me and I knew I wasn't going to get the job there and then. It wasn't a job I wanted anyway. The funny part came at the end of the interview:

Interviewer: "Thank you very much for coming, I'll show you out..."

Me: (wanting to walk around Television Centre) "No, no, you don't need to. I'll be fine, I know the way out."

The funny (and slightly eerie) thing was that I found myself walking round the circular corridor on my own. There was nobody else about. The corridor had lots of doors around it – I could have gone into any of them! I did see the *Breakfast with Frost* set.

Had I been there a bit later, I would have walked into *The Six O'Clock News*!

BBC Radio Solent in Southampton is another place I visited one Saturday. I spent the morning sitting in the studio with the guy who was driving the desk for Peter White (who is blind). In the afternoon, I watched what they did on their sports show – which was very interesting.

The station I wish I had made more effort to get into is BBC Southern Counties Radio. I wrote to and phoned them a few times but I wasn't persistent enough. Now, there is absolutely no doubt in my mind, had I been totally focussed and persistent, I would have got a job with the station This is how Gavin (at Surf) managed to get a job at that station – through sheer persistence. At the time, my mindset wasn't in a good state and I wasn't feeling confident.

Success in life is about desire. When you want something badly enough, the number one factor to achieving it is being persistent – and not giving up until you achieve what you really want.

If you would like proof of persistence, read *Think and Grow Rich* by Napoleon Hill. To give you an example, Mr WD (WD-40) only had to try thirty-nine incorrect formulas before he found the right solution.

In 1999, I went speed dating for the first time. I had to register online and, after the event, go online and tick the girls I liked for friendship or dating.

It was an evening event held in the basement of a restaurant, near to where Surf was. The most nerve-racking bit of the evening was arriving at the event and walking down the stairs because all of the people that were there then saw that I am disabled.

It surprised people. In mingling with people before the speed dating got started, some people spoke to me normally, whilst others were more reserved and patronising, saying "Alright mate..." and metaphorically patting me on the head.

There were twenty-five women and twenty-five guys and the organisers were helpful in changing the format of the speed dating. Normally, it's the women who stay seated whilst the guys move from table to table. The organisers swapped it around so that I didn't have to move.

The three minute speed dates weren't scary. With fifty conversations going on, it made it a really loud and hot environment. I had to make a real effort to sit forward and to speak very clearly. Most dates flew by and I would have liked more time to talk with each woman. While with a small number of women, we talked for a bit and then sat there, not knowing what else to say to each other, until the three minutes were up!

After the actual speed dating was finished, I went and spoke to the three or four women who I thought were nice.

One thing I find really physically difficult in life is speaking to someone while I'm standing up. I use so much energy standing up that I haven't got much energy left to speak. Over the course of about a year I went speed dating on three occasions and met up with one girl (Beverly) afterwards. That's a poor conversion rate of seventy-five to one.

At the time, people said to me something like, "You've only been speed dating three times. You haven't tried very hard." People don't understand (or think).

Going speed dating used up a tremendous amount of energy; walking from my car to the restaurant, walking down the stairs, standing around and talking to people, speaking clearly to twenty-people, more standing around and talking to people, walking up the stairs and back to my car. I use up four times as much energy than the average person – not only in walking but in speaking too.

However, after the speed dating, when nobody had selected me for friendship or dating, it took much more emotional energy out of me.

Speed dating is not the best way for me to find a girlfriend. It is unfortunate that my speech is affected by my CP because it is my speech which is a real turn off for most people. If my speech wasn't affected people would think *he just can't walk properly*.

Never have I liked being put in a 'disabled box' because I don't see myself as being disabled. Therefore, I've never wanted a disabled girlfriend. However, am I being a hypocrite? I don't know. I've always been of the opinion that having a girlfriend who is unable to walk properly would make my life physically harder.

It is something I'm sure some disabled people will disagree with me on. I remember discussing this with Martin and Janet years ago. We were of the opinion that two *severely* disabled people don't go together. Of course it is contentious thing to say and a grey area.

Consider this hypothetical scenario; a man and a woman who both walk with crutches have a baby. How do they carry the baby around?

Ultimately, it comes down to love and attraction. I am attracted to women who inspire me.

Oh yes – Beverly – the girl I met up with after speed dating. We spent four hours in a Brighton pub one Sunday afternoon chatting about everything under the sun. She seemed like a nice, down-to-earth girl. Towards the end of the afternoon, she said something that I thought was a bit strange. She said she wasn't ready to start a relationship because she had recently been attacked twice. I didn't ask her what sort of attacks she meant.

After giving Beverly a lift home from the pub, she texted me a few days later saying she had got home from a party where she had 'got off with a bloke'. Having met Beverly at a speed dating event, I thought it was a bit insensitive of her to tell me that. I didn't reply to her text message.

Over the years (mainly 2002-2011), I met so many women (mostly in pubs) and was no stranger to online dating.

Ever since I started to walk in 1984, people have been coming up to me in the street (seeing me walking or as I get in and out of my car) and have called me an inspiration. I always thank them, but over the years I have increasingly thought: *They have no idea what I do or the emotional pain I've been through – and have overcome.* Compared to my emotional struggles, physically, my life is a piece of cake.

I get the impression that most women just see me as being severely disabled. But I don't think or see myself as being a disabled person. In my mind, I'm a regular guy.

The most basic human emotion is love. Everyone needs to give and to receive love because it's the most fundamental thing in life. Also, one of the most natural things is to share life with someone.

When people see me walking around and doing everything I do, do they ever consider my basic needs and desires as a human being?

Not being physiologically fulfilled affects my confidence in everyday life. What really hurts me is, I have got so much love and affection to give. I'm such a soft and gentle guy, but people don't give me a chance and allow me to show them this side of me.

I think most people take relationships for granted (I've known so many people in bad relationships). It hurts me because I value people and relationships.

I often wonder how I keep going. It's due to my belief that I am going to find the right woman to share life with. I am only human.

While writing this book, I've heard Jeremy Vine on Radio 2 on his weekly series inviting an inspirational person into the studio to answer the question *"What makes us human?"* A few months ago, I heard Alison Lapper MBE (an English artist who paints with her mouth because she was born without any arms) on the programme. Alison defined it extremely well. She said, what makes us human is, "To love, to be loved, and to be accepted and respected."

In 1999, I started applying for IT jobs.

I heard about a scheme that Scope ran in partnership with some big companies such as McDonald's, offering a disabled person a twelve month placement on £12,000. I applied for it and got to the interview stage.

The interview process was a two day event, held somewhere that I drove to and stayed overnight. A couple of weeks beforehand, I was informed that I would have to do a five minute presentation on 'The role of the British Monarchy in the 21st century'. I felt like doing a five second presentation on it, saying they should all be made to go and live in council houses and fend for themselves! However, I did a bit of research.

The two day interview process wasn't enjoyable and I felt sick the whole time. There were five other people – all wheelchair-bound – going for a vacancy. It was strange, my feelings of worthlessness made me think they were all better than me. On the other hand, I knew that I was worth more than a temporary job on £12,000.

On the first day, my five minute presentation lasted ten minutes! In my defence, I am not the world's fastest speaker!

Then in the evening we all had to do activities together. However, during a break, someone overheard me throwing up in the toilet and the interviewers deemed that I wasn't good at working under pressure. I didn't see myself working for McDonald's in any case!

After catching a chest infection, Nan died in 1999. Clare phoned me with the news while I was putting petrol in my car, on my way to Surf. Hence, I went to Nan's home first.

Walking into her bedroom, there was Nan lying on her bed with Mum and Liz sitting on either side of the bed, stroking Nan's face. It felt odd and slightly morbid. Mum and Liz hadn't spoken to each other for about a year and they were talking quietly and stroking Nan's face. Nan just looked like she was asleep.

When I visited Nan towards the end of her life, visually, she recognised me but she had no idea who I was. She often thought that I was her brother. It became virtually impossible to have a conversation with her – so I just sat holding her hand for a while.

Coincidentally, Nan and Grandad both died aged eightynine from a chest infection. Nan was cremated in Brighton and her ashes were scattered in Shoreham.

At the time, Clare and I thought that Mum and Liz would forgive and forget, and make up but they didn't. Years later, they both met for a coffee when Liz had a cancer scare but they didn't connect.

Another sad thing that happened in 1999 was Neil (the manic depressive) got cancer (and died a year or two later).

On a happier note, in April that year, I went skiing in Aspen for two weeks. It came about through Carl (who was suing the family business at the time!). He was living in Aspen and was a volunteer at a disabled skiing school. Being on Income Support I was able to get a skiing scholarship. All I had to pay for were my flights, accommodation and food.

I flew to Denver and then onto Aspen in a smaller plane (due to Aspen having a short runway). On arriving in Aspen and walking out of the aircraft, the high altitude was immediately apparent as I had a slight shortness of breath. It wasn't a problem; I had my inhaler and soon acclimatised.

The ski resort (called Snowmass) had a bed and breakfast (where I stayed), and a few restaurants, bars and shops.

I went skiing every day and it was great fun. I skied in what I would describe as a one-man toboggan, which had two skis on the bottom of it and a long lead on the back of it. I always had an instructor with me, as well as a volunteer. To turn left or right I just leaned very slightly either side. At first, I was leaning too harshly but I soon got the hang of it.

The instructor skied behind me, holding the long lead, whilst the volunteer helped to lift my toboggan (with me in it) onto the ski lifts. There was an art to doing it, as the skilifts didn't stop!

Snowmass had various ski slopes, each having a name. The two names that I found hilarious were Fanny Hill and Sam's Knob! These names meant nothing to Americans.

There were a number of advanced disabled skiers at the resort who skied independently, using two ski sticks and with only one ski on the bottom of their toboggan.

Early one afternoon while skiing, I developed a really itchy rash all over my body. I went to the onsite medical centre, who gave me an injection in my arm. After the injection, I walked to the reception desk to pay my bill, at which point I fainted.

I would like to say that I fainted when I saw the size of my bill but it was due to the after effects of the injection (I've never been good when it comes to needles). The receptionist rushed round and grabbed me and they laid me on a bed for a few minutes until I was fine. It's a mystery what caused the rash but the injection quickly got rid of it.

Staying at the bed and breakfast I experienced something I have never experienced before, in all the places I've travelled to in the word (I don't know whether it was due to the high altitude).

Being my relaxed self on holiday, I got talking to an American family at breakfast. When they asked me where I was from, they could not understand me. It became embarrassing:

Me: "*England.*"

American lady: "India...? Indiana...?"

Me: "The UK."

American lady: "The Ukraine...?"

Saying, "London" or "Great Britain" didn't get through either.

Being my persistent self, I cracked it on the third morning. When the lady understood me saying "Europe" she then understood me saying "London." That's as close as I could be bothered to get!

It was very strange because the lady understood everything else I said. It made me think that due to my Cerebral Palsy, I probably don't have an English accent.

It felt like Groundhog Day! Writing about it now, it would have been easier to get a piece of paper and write *England* on it!

I recounted the ordeal to Jake, when I went to Maui again in 2002.

Me: "I don't have an English accent, do I?"

Jake: (in a very poor English accent) "I don't have an English accent..."

Then Jake said my accent does come through due to certain words and phrases that I use.

Back in Aspen, Carl came skiing with me a couple of times and we went into Aspen on a few occasions. He was a really good guy (and probably still is). We didn't talk about the pending court case much, as we both saw the funny side to it and how ridiculous it was.

The thing I didn't like about Aspen was wandering around in the evenings and having dinner on my own. I found it lonely and I wished I had a girlfriend. I felt like I was an outcast.

However, everyone I met on that trip was friendly and I had a good time in the bars I went to, talking to people. The really bizarre thing I found about Aspen was tipping the barman each time I bought a drink. I hadn't come across that before but it's customary in some parts of America.

Back at home in the summer of 1999, it was time for me to get a new car on Motability. I went for a Renault Mégane – and I've stuck with having a Mégane every time I've renewed my car. As the car has cruise control, I find it much easier to drive, and the keyless entry card thing is really handy. I don't need to take the key out of my pocket!

In 1999, I also started to look every week in the jobs section of the *Evening Argus*, Having already applied for a few jobs, in September I saw an IBM ad in the newspaper. The ad was promoting a graduate recruitment day in Leamington Spa. I registered to attend the event and drove up the day before, staying in a hotel overnight.

The following day (I think it was a Thursday) was pretty full on. It consisted of three interviews and three exam-like tests (known as the IBM IPAT). There were at least fifty graduates and we were split into groups. Although the three tests were all multiple choice, they were not easy, especially the third test, which included algebra/simultaneous equations, probability and fractions. I hadn't done that kind of maths since my first year of university, five years earlier.

Before the second and third tests started, the invigilator informed everyone that each correct answer was worth one mark and, to discourage people from guessing an answer, half a mark would be deducted for every wrong answer. The invigilator also advised people not to worry about answering every question, as nobody had ever completed the tests.

Calculators weren't allowed to be used in the tests. I had a problem because it took me a long time to handwrite the calculations, which only gave me enough time to answer a few of the questions.

At the end of the third test (I sound like a cricket commentator!), I went and spoke to the person in charge of the recruitment day, called Michael (he looked a bit like the main baddy from the film *Die Hard* – actor Alan Rickman).

In explaining the problem to Michael, I mentioned that at university I had had a scribe in my exams. Our conversation continued:

Michael: "Where do you live?"

Me: "I live near Brighton."

Michael: "Are you able to get to our head office in Portsmouth?"

Me: "Yes, that's not a problem."

Michael: (looking in his diary) "Can you make it on Tuesday of next week?"

Me: "Absolutely!"

Michael: "I will provide someone to scribe for you in order for you do the three tests. I'll also give you an interview on Tuesday morning as well. Will that be alright for you?"

Me: "That will be absolutely excellent. I can't believe it! I'm really pleased. Thank you very much for your help. I really appreciate it."

Michael: "You've very welcome and I look forward to seeing you on Tuesday."

Me: "Likewise!"

Michael was a real good guy!

I felt like I had really achieved something.

Having remained good friends with John Potts (JP) since university, I knew what I had to do when I got home from Leamington Spa, on that Thursday evening. I phoned JP, explained the situation and asked if there was any chance he could give me some maths tuition to refresh my memory on simultaneous equations, probability and fractions.

Reading this, you might be thinking that I had an unfair advantage. Maybe I did. What I know is that successful people seize opportunities in life.

Being the good guy that he is, JP and his housemate came to see me, from Hounslow, on Sunday. JP's housemate gave me more tuition than JP did that afternoon while JP caught up with my family! I didn't mind because they were both very good at refreshing memory with the maths I needed. JP and his housemate really helped me.

After three hours of slightly heavy maths coaching my brain felt a bit frazzled. But I was feeling confident and excited about Tuesday. I was excited because IBM were giving me the opportunity to show them how intelligent I was (and am).

When I arrived at IBM on Tuesday morning, I first had a forty-five minute interview (discussion) with Michael. It included him testing out my logical mind; by asking me to list verbally the things I had done that morning, from getting out of bed to arriving at IBM.

Everything I listed, Michael wrote on a whiteboard.

He then asked me to breakdown how I got to Portsmouth. I replied. "By driving my car," and I listed all of the main roads I went on.

His next question was, "Specifically, how did you find our head office?" My answer included pulling over when I got to Chichester to look at my print-out of AutoRoute directions, looking at signposts when I got to Portsmouth, and pulling over to ask someone walking past when I got near to IBM.

Michael seemed happy with my logic. Being an analytical person, I found that exercise easy and fun!

After a coffee break, I did the first test with Laura, who scribed the things I asked her to write down in order for me to work out the answers to questions. Laura was one of the nicest young ladies that I have met in life (in every sense!).

The first test was all about logic. Although I wouldn't describe the test as being easy, it wasn't too bad. And because no points were deducted for wrong answers on this test, I answered all of the questions.

After lunch, it was time for test number two. It was on sequences and working out what the next item in the sequence was. It wasn't sequences of numbers, it was sequences of letters.

I came prepared for the test by having a piece of paper, on which I'd printed the letters of the alphabet and numbering them one to twenty-six. It made it easier to convert the letters into numbers and then work out the sequences.

You may think the second test wasn't that difficult but, like all of the three tests, it got progressively harder – especially once each item in the sequences became double letters – and then triple letters!

I didn't answer all of the questions in test two because I didn't want to risk getting an answer wrong and thus losing half a mark.

However, I spent a long time, trying my best, going over the questions I didn't initially answer and working out the answer to some of them, that by the time I had finished the second test it was four o'clock. Laura, therefore, asked me to come back in two days to do the third test!

Michael and Laura weren't concerned with how much time I took to do the second test. It was obvious to Laura that I wanted to do my best and that I didn't want to give up. Needless to say IBM were very accommodating.

Felling tired, I was pleased with my performance on the first two tests. I knew the third one was a stinker.

There were forty questions in test three – and I spent all of that Thursday on it. I first answered all of the questions that I was confident about. Then I went back over the harder questions.

One of the easier questions was about a leaking swimming pool, which stated how much water leaked every twenty-four hours and gave the dimensions of the pool. The question was something like 'How much water would you need to put in every hour to keep the pool six eighths full?'

A lot of the questions involved me asking Laura to write down long and tedious calculations, which I had to work out.

In the afternoon I was becoming frustrated because the questions were so difficult. Laura was really encouraging, saying things like, "Come on Patrick, I know you can do this one..."

In the end, I answered thirty-one of the forty questions.

Most of the remaining nine questions I had narrowed down to two of the five multiple choice answers – but I didn't want to chance losing half a mark by taking a guess at the answer. I went over the nine questions three or four times. I was so determined to succeed.

The third IBM IPAT test is the most mentally taxing thing I have ever done. I put everything I had into it.

I remember sitting in my car, in the IBM car park at 4.30 pm, feeling absolutely mentally and physically drained. I felt sick due to being so exhausted. I don't know how I managed to drive home from Portsmouth that day. My overwhelming feeling of having done well probably helped.

The following week I received a phone call from Laura to congratulate me. She said I had done extremely well in all three IPAT tests and that they were very impressed with me.

She continued by saying they were happy to accept me, and my acceptance letter would be in the post (which is now in my filing cabinet!), and my starting salary would be £16,000, once they had found me a role (in computing).

Needless to say, I felt elated. Was it my biggest achievement so far in life?

Laura asked me if I would be happy to work in their head office in Portsmouth. I said I wasn't sure but that I would think about it and get back to her in the next few days.

It had only been a couple of weeks since I had seen the IBM ad in the newspaper for the recruitment day in Leamington Spa. I wasn't expecting to be in this position.

On the one hand, I was overjoyed with my awesome achievement and with the prospect of working for IBM. It helped me to overcome my feeling of worthlessness. On the other hand, the thought of having to move to Portsmouth terrified me. I was still very weak emotionally.

When I phoned Laura back I was noncommittal. I didn't say no to working in Portsmouth but I said I would rather work closer to home. I asked her if there was an IBM office in Brighton. Laura didn't say there wasn't one. She said she would look to see what she could find and get back to me.

In a way I wish Laura had said to me that I had to work in their head office. Moving to Portsmouth would have given me the kick up the ass I needed – it would have done me the world of good.

I am not sure what happened over the next month or so (October/November) but I think Laura moved onto another role in IBM herself and my case was passed onto someone who hadn't met me. I kept phoning and chasing IBM every couple of weeks, they just said they were still looking for a role for me.

Sometime in 1999, Clare and I both received a letter from Dad, that included some photos. The letter was to inform us that he had got married to a Moroccan Muslim girl (called Madeline), who is the same age as me. The photos were of Dad and Madeline getting married. Needless to say, Clare and I were a bit surprised and shocked.

At the beginning of December 1999 we (Clare, Rupert, Scott, Oliver, Mum and I – as well as a couple with two small kids who were friends with Clare and Rupert), went on a two week holiday to St Lucia, where Clare and Rupert got married.

It was the worst holiday I have been on. Mum was an absolute nightmare, due to her non-acceptance of the marriage. I remember Clare saying that Mum had ruined her wedding day.

We all stayed in a three star all-inclusive resort. The weather was very hot and the staff were really nice. I took a particular liking to one of the St Lucian waitresses!

The resort was quite big and spread out, which meant I was in my wheelchair most of the time. The place was fairly wheelchair accessible but it meant having to go a long way round to use the ramps.

As I've mentioned before, due to my poor coordination I have never found it easy to push myself in my wheelchair. Pushing myself up long slopes is tremendously difficult – and it's on the verge of being impossible – hence why people often help me up hills. The hot weather also made me feel lethargic.

Also as you know by now, spending much time in my wheelchair tightens up my hamstrings and gives me a numb bum!

For most people, going on holiday to an all-inclusive resort is a relaxing time. For me, it's a time when I use a lot of energy just to get around. Still, it has never stopped me from going on holiday.

Without meaning do so now, I've kind of listed the reasons why I hate (and I don't use the word lightly) using my wheelchair. However, what I hate the most about being in a wheelchair is people having to physically look down at me.

The world is full of steps and stairs, I cannot imagine life without being able to walk up and down them.

Anyway, back in St Lucia – whenever I've stayed in a resort on holiday, being my relaxed sociable self, I meet and chat to loads of people and somehow I become infamous around the resort. As was the case in St Lucia.

Wandering around in my wheelchair, I saw four local elderly guys playing backgammon with each other. After watching them play for a while, from a distance, I wheeled myself up to them and asked if I could play.

I'm sure they thought I was a bit stupid at first. However, their minds soon changed after I had beaten the four of them, one after the other! Backgammon is a game I don't often play but never forget.

All the while on holiday, I was still hopeful that IBM were going to find me a role (albeit not feeling as confident as I had been).

Mum's friend, Mary, (one of our neighbours in Belgium and who now lived in America) came to stay at the resort, for two or three days for Clare and Rupert's wedding which was held at the end of the first week of our holiday.

Apart from a tropical rainstorm in the morning – and Mum showing her disapproval of the pending wedding, by her not-so-secret conversations with Mary – the wedding ceremony went fine (although I recall Clare fainting briefly at one point due to the stress or the heat).

In order for Clare and Rupert to have a week without Scott and Oliver, it was planned that Mum, the two boys and I would spend the second week at Club Med, on the other side of St Lucia.

However, with Mum still feeling very vexed about the new marriage, she was moaning and swearing at me, in front of Scott and Oliver (who were only three and one). I was finding the situation so stressful and upsetting that I was retching and vomiting in front of the three of them (which was something that I rarely did in front of people). It caused Mum to shout at me – which just made me feel worse.

I lasted at Club Med for three days before I went back to the first resort we stayed at. Clare moaned at me at the end of the holiday because she said I didn't do much when I returned to the first resort. The weather was extremely hot and I wanted to leave Clare and Rupert to themselves

Back home, in early 2000, I received the letter from IBM that I had been hoping wouldn't arrive. It said that, unfortunately, they had been unable to find me a suitable role and, because they didn't like to keep people holding on for too long, they weren't looking to employ me anymore. I tried phoning Michael several times but I never got through to him.

It was deeply disappointing and it diminished my confidence again. However it was a good thing. The acceptance letter I received from IBM helped me to get a better job with another large corporation in 2001.

I was still working at Surf but, by the turn of the new millennium, I was only going into the radio station a couple of days per week.

Rarely would I vomit somewhere else other than at home. However, during the two and a half years at Surf, my feeling of worthlessness became so deep that I threw up in the production studio on two occasions.

One time I managed to be sick into the wastepaper bin, which I discretely went to wash out in the toilet sink. Ironically the bin had a hole in the middle of the bottom of it – therefore I had to carry the bin at an angle so that the vomit didn't fall out via the hole.

On the other occasion, I was a bit sick on the production studio carpet – which I quickly cleaned up – but people knew that I had been sick. I beat myself up about that episode for several days afterwards.

In early 2000, things weren't good; I hadn't got a job at IBM, I wasn't happy at Surf, or at home, Mum was constantly going on at me about how her life was so hard and unfair, with everyone against her, whilst at the same time saying that I wasn't trying hard enough in life and that I needed to get a proper job.

My vomiting was out of control. I couldn't take it anymore. I needed to get some help.

The first therapist I went to wasn't good for me because she made me feel really anxious. I remember sitting on her couch and retching, as if I was going to be sick. Worryingly, her way of dealing with the situation was to shout at me slightly, in an authoritative manner: "Don't be sick here. You can't be sick here. It is not allowed..." It made me think that she was an idiot! I only went to her the once.

Maggie, the second therapist was good. She practised Cognitive Behavioural Therapy (CBT). I must have gone to Maggie one morning a week for about six months, during which time she answered some of the things that I didn't understand and that had been troubling me, including why in nightclubs I was often approached by gay men.

Maggie said to me, "You are a severely disabled young man and therefore gay men see you as easy prey and an easy target."

Once Maggie had said that, it didn't faze me anymore. Although I understood what Maggie meant, I thought, *I'm not that disabled,*

Since then, when I've been in a pub or club and have occasionally been approached by a gay man, I remain calm and get a member of staff to deal with whoever keeps on annoying me. Let me tell you, I am not easy prey!

Back on Maggie's couch, I discussed the molestation event at boarding school. Ironically, Maggie explained that it was perfectly normal for boys aged between seven and thirteen to play and experiment with each other sexually.

Without me ever mentioning my friendship with Nathan to Maggie, she helped me get over something that had been troubling me for sixteen years! It caused me to Google, and read up on, 'childhood sexual experimentation' – and that is how I overcame what happened with Nathan.

(As I have already mentioned, I think that being the new boy at middle school, and slowly walking around the playground with my rollator also had something to do with it.)

However, at fifteen or sixteen, Maggie explained that what happened with Freddie at boarding school was more like abuse and that Freddie might have seen me as an easy target.

Most of the time with Maggie was spent with her trying to change the negative thoughts I had about myself into positive thoughts. She advised me to go home and write a series of positive statements about myself and to stick them on my bedroom wall.

Every week when I arrived home from seeing Maggie, Mum (who was working from home), ALWAYS asked me, "How was your therapy?"

It REALLY annoyed me and I felt like replying, "It's none of your business." But saying that would start an argument – so I ALWAYS replied, "Alright." Mum only accused me of grunting at her then.

When I wrote positive statements about myself, on my computer in my bedroom and stuck them on my wall, Mum often came in and passed her judgement on what I was doing. She referred to the positive statements as my 'affirmations'.

Living with my mother I felt I had no space or privacy.

Maggie made me feel good about myself – but every week when I got home – I felt bad again.

Writing about it now, I find it really strange that I don't remember talking to Maggie much about the relationship I had with my mother. I think, being in the situation I was in, I was too close to the problem to see it. Also, I felt I wasn't succeeding in helping Mum to take some responsibility for herself – which made me feel that I wasn't trying hard enough. It was a horrible situation to be in.

Several times over the years, when I suggested to Mum that having counselling would do her good, she always replied something like, "I don't need counselling, there's nothing wrong with me."

While seeing Maggie I became more focussed again on finding a job in IT. Having not done any computer programming since university (where I learnt Ada, which was quite an old language even at that time), I thought it would be a good idea if I learnt an up-to-date language. Speaking to my friend Stuart, who was a Foxpro database programmer, we ascertained that Visual Basic 6 (VB) was a good language to learn.

I bought a good step-by-step, three to four hundred page, book (which came with VB installation CDs) – and over no more than four months I taught myself VB.

Although I found the step-by-step book slow, it suited my learning style and I went through the first half of it quickly. I found VB straightforward.

Once I reached about halfway through the book, I wrote a little animation program that blew a puff of smoke out of a chimney of a house, which rose up to the top of the computer screen.

This gave me the idea of writing 'a bat and ball' game (similar to the tennis game that plugged into the television which I played with Douglas at Mary's house in the early 1980s in Belgium).

I felt I knew enough VB syntax to write the game – and just used the book as reference guide to look things up from then on.

I added more and more features to the game as I built it, such as increasing the speed of the ball by 10% every time it hit the bat (which was controlled using the mouse), giving the player an extra life when they accumulated certain points, getting the player to enter their name, which enabled their highest score to be written to, and retrieved from, a file.

I also made the game really colourful, as I thought Scott would like to play it, which he did (for a couple of days!).

In writing the game, I taught myself a lot of VB. I felt it was a real achievement.

In my experience, all you need to be a good programmer is to be logically minded and good at problem solving. The most important thing is knowing how to debug a program (step through the code line by line). Once you can do that, it becomes easy to pick up the syntax and see what's going on.

As I got myself back into computers, I thought it would be fun and interesting to go to a computing and robotics exhibition in London – which I went to by train.

When I arrived at the conference centre, I took the lift upstairs in my wheelchair. The lift was small and looked very new. It wasn't much fun when the lift got stuck between two floors!

In pressing the alarm button, a lady came to the bottom of the lift and said to me that they were going to call an engineer out to free me. Although the lady stayed and chatted to me, I was stuck in the lift for forty minutes – in which time I hatched a cunning plan!

When the engineer arrived and had unstuck the lift, most people would just be grateful and relieved to have been let out of the lift.

Lift engineer: "Sorry it's taken me so long to get here. I've come from the other side of London."

Me: Thank you very much, I really appreciate it."

Then he said something which was really going to help me!

Lift engineer: (mainly addressing the lady) "This lift should not be open to the public yet. It was only fitted three days ago and it hasn't been serviced yet."

Me: (addressing the lady, politely but authoritatively) "I'm really not happy. How can this happen? I want to see the centre manager and make a complaint."

The lady took me up (in another lift!) to a series of posh offices and into the centre manager's office. I felt very confident – because I had nothing to lose.

I politely had a little rant at the manager:

Me: "I felt really scared and claustrophobic stuck in that small lift. Why is the lift open to the public when it hasn't been serviced yet?"

After the manager appeared to be very apologetic:

Me: (authoritatively) "I would like some financial compensation..."

Manager: "How much are you thinking of?"

Me: (thinking for a couple of seconds) "Two hundred pounds."

Manager: (after a slight pause) "I can arrange that for you."

I then wished I had asked for more money!

Manager: "I'll get my PA to take you for lunch while I sort out a cheque for you."

After having a free lunch with a nice girl (in the cafeteria), she took me back up to the manager's office. I signed a waiver (not to take the matter any further) and the manager gave me a cheque for £200.

I then went and really enjoyed the exhibition!

In early summer of 2000, after two years at Surf I was given the opportunity that I had been waiting for. The three daytime presenters where going to have a team meeting outside of the radio station. Jason, who was the drivetime presenter, decided to record some dry links and let me playout the whole show.

By then, *The List* was a twenty-five minute magazine show of the past – hence drivetime was 3.00 to 7.00 pm.

After playing-out the first two links, I relaxed and the entire show went extremely well. It was a good programme to do because after 4.00 pm there were news bulletins and traffic/travel updates every half hour.

The traffic/travel news was provided by an external company, who dialled up the station's ISDN line (an ISDN is like a high quality phone line). I don't recall Surf having a talkback facility in order to speak to the person on the ISDN off-air. It was just a case of checking to hear if the travel guy had dialled up, playing the travel jingle and putting the ISDN fader up.

One at a time, I loaded one of Jason's pre-recorded links onto a touch-screen button and played it over the end/start of a song. It was so easy and fun.

Having done such a good job of playing-out a drivetime show, I felt I had proved myself. Had I had something else to go to, I think I would have left Surf at that point.

Shortly after I had done drivetime, Jason had to cover a Sunday breakfast show for the regular presenter. Rather than having to get up earlier to present the show live, Jason pre-recorded the links and got me to play the show out. I wasn't at all pleased with how that show went, however.

The Sunday breakfast show was 7.00 to 11.00 am. I was used to going into the station on my own at the weekends and, on that Sunday, wanted to get there early so I could take my time making my flask of coffee, walking up the stairs and to get everything set up in the production studio.

Arriving at the front of Surf at 6.00 am, I was expecting to be able to open the door with my key fob, as I normally would do. However, somebody had locked a second lock, which I didn't have a key to.

What do I do? What do I do? I thought, and then phoned Jason. After moaning that I had woken him up, Jason said he would come and let me in. Having given him a lift home from the pub before I knew he only lived a five minute walk away. Nevertheless, I asked him to hurry up a bit, as I was standing outside in the rain.

After waiting for twenty minutes I was quite agitated. After twenty-five minutes I phoned Jason. He answered the phone sounding half asleep and said "Oh, I fell back to sleep..."

It infuriated me and I said, "I'll come and get the key from you."

Rushing back to my car and over to Jason's place, he walked out of his flat bleary-eyed and he couldn't get the key I needed off of his key ring. Authoritatively, I said, "Give me all of your keys, I haven't got time for this."

It was 7.35 am by the time I had got everything set up in the production studio. I hadn't made any coffee and just had some water as I went past the kitchen area. I had rushed so fast into the building and up the stairs that I felt like I had nearly given myself a heart attack.

The show went fine but I hadn't enjoyed it. During the show I asked myself "Why am I doing this?"

Having got up at 5.00 am, after not much sleep, I had expended a tremendous amount of energy – and was doing something for free that I wasn't enjoying. It felt like utter madness and perhaps one step beyond a joke.

After having had a coffee, once the show was over, I phoned Jason and made him come to the radio station to get his keys – where I gave him a piece of my mind.

The following is a deeply personal event, which also has a funny side to it. (I don't remember exactly when it took place but I know I was twenty-six.)

For months (and years) I had been thinking about going to a prostitute. I had got as far as getting a number of cards from a phone box in Brighton and trying to pluck up the courage to phone one of them. However, after a few weeks I thought it was uncool to be driving my car around, with prostitute cards in my glove box – so I threw them away in a public bin.

Then, one Thursday in 2000, after an absolutely unbelievable argument with Mum, I decided not to go home that evening. Instead, I was going to sleep on the sofa, in the reception area at Surf.

After getting a burger to eat quite late that evening, on the spur of the moment, I decided I was going to go to a prostitute.

I went to the same phone box as before and picked the card which said something like 'Slim and sexy dark-haired female – central Brighton'.

Standing up in the phone box, feeling very nervous, I called the number on the card. After a lady answered the phone, and me hyperventilating for a few seconds:

Lady: "Do you want the address of where we are?"

Me: "Yeah."

Fortunately, not being very good at map-reading, I knew the street where I was going to – and it was a basement flat.

Surprisingly, after putting the phone down, my mind went into the present moment; I was feeling quite confident and thinking very clearly.

I drove over and found somewhere to park nearby. After walking down the stairs and ringing the bell, I was greeted by the lady I had spoken to on the phone. She was in her forties or fifties and the madam of the flat!

After speaking to her about what I wanted, I asked her if I could pay with my Visa Debit card! She replied no.

Now, don't ask me why I thought I could pay for sex with a prostitute using my debit card. Even I find it bizarre. I obviously wasn't thinking that clearly!

I asked the lady what time they closed. With there being only about an hour until closing time, I said, "I'll go get some cash and I'll be back."

I pegged it up the stairs, back to my car and rushed over to a side street, where I knew there was an ATM. After getting cash and back in my car, I wanted to turn right out of the side street but it had a 'no right turn' sign. It was past 11 o'clock and there was no traffic about – so I thought, *fuck it* and turned right.

The next thing I saw was a police car behind me, flashing its blue light! Since leaving the prostitute, I had been thinking, *hurry up, the brothel closes at midnight*. Remember, I was in the present moment and I was full of adrenaline.

I pulled over, opened my window and waited for the policeman. On arriving at my car door, he said, "What have you just done?"

This is what went through my mind: *Well, it depends, how long you have been following me? I've been to a prostitute and tried to pay for sex using my debit card. Then I've been to get cash and now I'm going back to the prostitute.*

However, I innocently replied, "What do you mean?"

Policeman: "You turned right out of a road, where it is clearly signposted not to do so..."

Me: "I'm really sorry, it's late at night and there was no traffic about. So I thought it was safe to do so..."

The policeman let me go after a minute or two and I made it back to the basement flat. After paying the madam the cash, I was led into a room, which had a voluptuous double bed in it, and where I met the prostitute.

She gave me a little 'menu card' and we spoke about what I wanted. I didn't need the menu card because I knew what I wanted. As I had already said to the madam, I wanted to have intercourse.

Then the prostitute left the room for me to get undressed. Although the bed was quite high, I was still full of adrenaline and it didn't take me long to get undressed.

The prostitute was fairly attractive but when she came back into the room her attitude had changed completely. She made it totally obvious that she wasn't too enamoured about having sex with me. Had the prostitute gone out of the room to say to the madam that she didn't want to go through with it?

First, we had a little disagreement about which position to adopt. Her favourite phrase seemed to be, "Oh for fuck's sake..."

Can anyone imagine how I felt?

I couldn't believe it. The adrenaline high I had quickly disappeared and I felt worthless again.

After having not very enjoyable sex for a few minutes, she passed me a couple of tissues.

As I sat myself up on the edge of the bed, she said, "Can you throw the condom in the bin over there (pointing to the far right corner of the room). Before we had started, she put my crutches in the left corner of the room – out of my reach.

Me: "How do you expect me to get to the bin? If you pass me my crutches I'll do it."

Prostitute: "Oh for fuck's sake..." (as she went and got the bin).

Then, it was time to get dressed. However, the bed was too high for me to put one foot on the floor, in order to balance myself.

There I was naked, lying on my back, with my right leg up in the air and my sock in my left hand, trying to reach my right foot. It would have taken me all night to get dressed.

Me: "I am really sorry to ask you but the bed is too high for me to get myself dressed. Please can you help me?"

Prostitute: "Oh for fuck's sake..."

I wasn't too enamoured with the situation either.

Ironically, there was a small ghetto blaster in the corner of the room (by the bin), playing weird ambient music. It was Surf!

We didn't say another word to each other. When I was dressed she let me out of the flat.

It was the most humiliating experience. Not what I had hoped for, for my first time. But I'm pleased I had the guts to do it.

The prostitute hadn't helped my self-esteem issues or my feeling of worthlessness. It took me months to rationalise her negative attitude towards me; she was quite young and I may have been her first disabled client.

I went back to Surf and was on one of the computers downstairs when, at about ten to one, the freelance presenter, who was on air, came running down the stairs in a bit of a panic. It was his first show and nobody had told or shown him what to do at the end of his show. I think he thought that at 1 o'clock, some music would magically start to play!

I went upstairs and showed him how to open the day's music log into a playlist.

After a few uncomfortable hours dozing on the sofa, at about 5.30 am, the breakfast presenter and the morning news guy arrived, who were surprised to see me there.

As we got on well, the news guy came over shortly after and asked me if I was okay. Without going into any detail, I said I had had a bad argument with Mum and that I had been to a prostitute – to which he replied, "Good on you mate!"

I haven't told anyone else about my liaison with the prostitute – until now!

Sill at Surf, Kevin, who was one of the volunteers who did a lot of production work at the station, also presented a seventies and eighties disco show on Saturday evening. As Kevin wasn't too keen to work on Saturday evenings, in mid to late August, we organised that he would pre-record the links for the show and I would play it out.

It was a fun and easy two hour show to do – and I was invoicing Surf £25 a week for playing out the programme. I did the show for three or four weeks, until Kevin found out and complained that I was getting paid for doing it, at which point Surf said to me, "We can't pay you anymore for playing- out the show."

I replied, "Okay, I'm not doing it anymore then."

I had achieved my goal!

It's funny because at the time, I thought Kevin was getting paid to present the show, but writing about it now, I don't think he was.

Over the last the four years, a few people have asked me if I believe in fate – I don't know. Maybe I do, because of what happened next.

In mid-September 2000, while looking through the *Evening Argus* jobs section, I spotted an advertisement for a course with the Prince's Trust. The advert read something like 'Are you 18 to 25? Would you like to do a 12-week course to help you get back into work?'

Although I was twenty-six, I thought, *there's no harm in phoning up* – so I did.

I spoke to Gemma, who was running the course, explained my circumstances and said I would like to find a job as a computer programmer. She asked me if I could go and meet her at the Prince's Trust office in Hove.

When I met Gemma, she told me a bit about the course which sounded too vocational for me. It sounded like it was intended for people who had been in prison and for recovering drug addicts. I didn't think it was for me.

However, Gemma wanted me to do it because she said I would inspire the people on the course. She seemed like a very genuine person and said if I did the course, she would do her best to help me find a job at the end of it. I couldn't refuse – it was a win/win situation.

The timing was a bit spooky. The last show that I playedout on Surf was on Saturday, 16th September. I emailed Jason during the following week, saying I was leaving and my last day at the station was on Friday 22nd September. I started the Prince's Trust course on the following Monday (25th September 2000).

Using my initiative – phoning up to find out more about the Prince's Trust course – resulted with a life-changing outcome (getting a good job). Imagine you were twenty-six years old and looking for a job – if you had seen an advert which started 'Are you between 18 and 25?', would you have phoned up about that opportunity?

I walked out of Surf with my head held high. However, emotionally, I was dishevelled. I felt like I was on my knees. It felt like I had put myself through hell to achieve my goal at Surf.

It was odd, unlike in the past when I have achieved something, achieving this goal, didn't bring me any joy. Maybe it's because I never told anyone about the goal that I had set myself. Maybe it's because not many people at the station respected me. Maybe it's because I didn't get any recognition for what I had achieved.

In leaving the station I took my little desk – but I left my chair. The chair had been so used and abused by people that it resembled my emotional state.

The good thing about it was I proved to myself that, with enough desire and self-belief, I can achieve anything I want to in life.

What drives me in life (apart from my Renault Mégane on cruise control) is *doing the impossible* – to achieve extraordinary things which I know I can do – but which some people have told me I would not be able to achieve. I have always felt the need to prove myself and show people what I can do. I think it has been partly so that people will accept me.

Upon writing this book, I continue to be a very driven person. However, I no longer feel the need to prove myself to people.

Chapter 10

As you can see, it's nearly the end of this book! As I said in the Introduction, when I had finished writing my autobiography (in May 2014) and mentioned to Stephanie Hale (my publishing adviser) that it was 216,000 words, she replied "That's too many words for one book, I suggest splitting it into two books."

Therefore, these are some of the things you can look forward to reading in the sequel!

- How I got a temporary job at the fire brigade – and then
- went onto work for a corporate company in IT.
- Buying and moving into my flat.
- Working for another radio station, producing the Saturday
- afternoon sports show for nine years.
- How I became a Saturday night DJ in a busy and popular
- pub.
- How I met lots of women.
- In 2009, Clare went through a messy and painful separation
- with her husband. Emotionally, it affected the
- family and I was the only one who was able to support
- Clare, financially, for six months. I also advised her on
- how to cope emotionally with the separation.
- In 2010, how I got into property investment, which
- triggered the journey that I'm now on.
- Deciding to take a change and leave my 'job for life'.
- How I persuaded my employer to make me redundant.
- They didn't want to do so and they thought I was mad!
- Purchasing two buy-to-let properties. Going into property
- investment was a turning point for me – and the
- best thing I have done so far in life. Whilst working tremendously
- hard over the last five years, it has also been

- an amazing voyage of discovery.

I have learnt so much:

- About people, human behaviour and psychology.
- Many different recursive strategies of making money
- from property (a recursive strategy is something that
- you can repeat an infinite number of times).
- The importance that maintaining a good mindset has
- on being successful.
- The Law of Attraction and the difference between
- pushing and pulling (this in itself was a turning point
- because it made me decide to stop going out to look for
- a girlfriend).

At the beginning of my journey, I thought, I am going to make £1 million, I've just got to find the right property strategy which suits me.

I started writing a blog and began networking in the property investment community. Ever since I started going to property networking events, people have called me an inspiration. At first, I found it really strange because I thought, I'm just a regular guy, what have I done? I haven't achieved anything yet.

The final thing I had to do was detach myself from my family. It stopped the stress and pain they were causing me.

Another discovery that I have found, as a result getting into property, is my purpose in life: To help and inspire people – and to reach my full potential.

I realised I have a gift in life – I inspire people just by doing the things that I do. It's a great gift to possess.

Since getting into property investment, my ambition has altered. At first, I had the idea of making £1 million – because I understand the process and relished the challenge. However, I'm not a materialistic person – £1 million is just an eye-catching figure that I thought of. What I love doing is speaking about mindset success and inspiring people. Stairs For Breakfast is giving me a platform as a public speaker.

I have learnt so many things about success and human behaviour in the last few years. Here are some of them.

Everyone creates their own reality (and perception). For example, I could think that my life is too difficult, and I could decide to give up and go and live in a residential home for disabled people. Instead, I have always thought, I can do anything I want to in life.

My main motivation for writing Stairs For Breakfast is because I want to inspire people and have decided to make a difference in the world.

Everyone has the power to choose how they live their life. Ultimately, it comes down to the thoughts you have about yourself (and about other people) and the decisions you make.

Reciprocity – let me ask you this question: has someone done you a favour or helped you out, when you then felt the need to return the favour by helping them in some way? This is reciprocity.

If you would like help from someone, help them first, without expecting anything in return, and then (most) people will help you in abundance.

I find it interesting that I learnt about reciprocity at the age of twelve, when I went to the local shops in my wheelchair.

Another reason for helping people is because it's virtually impossible to know how (or have the time or money) to do everything yourself. This is why people in property investment joint venture (work together).

By networking and meeting so many people in property who inspire me, I find that inspiration works both ways. I first had the idea of writing an autobiographical book in late 2010. I thought about it for two and a half years, before I began to write it.

Two people in the property investment community who stand out a proverbial mile for me are Paul Ribbons and Glenn Armstrong. They have both taught, helped and inspired me so much over the last five years – without me asking them for help. The thing which makes me feel so humble is, they both really want me to succeed.

I often refer to Paul as being like a dad to me. However, with Paul being eleven or twelve years older than me, he would rather I thought of him more like a brother! I couldn't wish for a better mentor than Glenn.

Paul inspired me to start writing my autobiography when he advised me: "Include everything in the book because it's a way of wiping the slate clean."

Shortly afterwards, Glenn asked me to send him a synopsis of my book – and then came back with, "At the end of every day, email me how many words you've written."

I did what Glenn advised. Every day, for the following fifteen months, I emailed Glenn a word count, until I had finished writing my autobiography. It took me fifteen months to write 216,000 words. On average I wrote between 700 and 1,000 per day. I typed every word with my left index finger. When you have enough desire and self-belief you can achieve anything in life.

Writing the autobiography has really helped me.

The only painful part of the book was writing about Rosie in Chapter 6. However, speaking to Paul and the CBT exercise I went through at the end of the chapter, really helped me. At the time (over eighteen months ago), Paul said to me something that is so true: "You are choosing to feel the way you do at the moment." Chapter 7 was a bit difficult to write, but the pain I was still feeling dissipated during Chapter 8. Then, during writing Chapter 9, I realised that I no longer felt bad about the letter I sent to Rosie in 1993.

At around the same time (autumn 2013) Glenn sent me an A4-sized inspirational poster, containing many lines, such as:

This is your life.

Do what you love, and do it often.

If you don't like something, change it.

Open your mind, arms and heart to new things.

The line which resonates with me the most is:

If you are looking for the love of your life, stop; they will be waiting for you when you start doing things you love.

You can find the poster online by searching for: *'this is your life poster'*.

It helped me to become at peace with myself. All I'm doing now is being my natural self and doing the things I love.

One of my passions is speaking about mindset success. *(Success = 95% Mindset + 5% Action)*

Something I've learnt a bit about is how the mind works; I find it interesting.

One of the main jobs of the mind is to protect us. It acts like our defence mechanism and therefore it is constantly looking for potential dangers. The mind is also like a library; storing all of our (harmful) experiences throughout life and thus, when it comes across a similar harmful situation, or what it perceives could lead to a similar harmful situation, the mind alerts us: "Danger, I don't like this... ". This is one of the reasons why people have so many negative thoughts.

It is said that all fears and phobias are derived from past experiences and learnt behaviours.

The mind loves having problems to solve because it keeps it occupied. The mind is also highly critical of the things we do (some people refer to it as our *inner voice*).

In the book *The Power of Now* by Eckhart Tolle, he talks about how to become *the watcher* of the mind's thoughts. This is how I got into Ascension Meditation – because it helps you become very aware of your thoughts, and teaches how to become present (live in the present moment). It requires practice and commitment but it's well worth it.

At a property networking event in 2011, I saw a demonstration of what happens to a human's mind in life. It was such a powerful presentation (analogy), I am going to describe it for you now.

The elements of the demonstration were:
- A glass jug of pure water.
- Bucket loads of water – representing positive experiences
- (and thoughts).
- A syringe containing brown dye – representing negative
- experiences (and thoughts).

As we go through life, we face a series of positive and negative experiences. In this demonstration, the contents of the jug represent the human mind.

Picture this:

When a baby is born, its mind is pure – *the glass jug of pure water.*

Then, at some point, the person has a negative experience – a few drops of brown dye are squirted into the jug and the water becomes slightly murky and unclear.

Then the person experiences something positive – quite a bit of water (from one of the buckets) is poured into the jug (the jug overflows) and the contents of the jug become a bit clearer.

Throughout the person's life, as negative and positive experiences (and thoughts) occur, more brown dye is squirted into the jug, and bucketloads of water are poured into the jug.

Note: relationally, bucketloads of water are needed to purify the contents of jug, once it has been intoxicated with only a small amount of brown dye.

It is said you become the average of the people you surround yourself with. That's why it's important to surround yourself with positive and successful people.

Remember: Success = 95% Mindset + 5% Action.

Writing my autobiography has been the most enduring – and also, the most satisfying – thing I think I've ever done.

Over the course of writing the autobiography, one of the things I've realised about myself relates to the time after moving back from Belgium in 1984, living in the second- floor flat.

In Chapter Three, I described that short period as being happy and sunny and mentioned the three songs which remind me of that time. It wasn't until I was writing the second half of my autobiography (the sequel) when I realised the significance of what I have written in Chapter Three.

I realised that happy time in 1984 was the last time that I was truly happy. It made me realise that I have been unhappy for the last thirty years.

All I can say now is, it doesn't matter anymore because I have overcome all of the dark experiences in my life. Pretty much everything that I have achieved over the last thirty years, I've done in a state of unhappiness.

Since getting into property investment, I have often said and thought, *I've only used 10% of my full potential so far.* It makes my mind boggle when I think about what I can achieve now that I am happy. It's amazing!

As for the future – I don't know what *Stairs For Breakfast* is going to lead to – I'm on an amazing journey! All I want to do now is promote my book and inspire people.

Recently, I did a book talk in front of twenty people. I was feeling slightly nervous beforehand, but once I started, I found myself in the present moment and in my element! I had considered creating a Powerpoint presentation and decided not to.

My 'off the top of my head' talk was excellent. I spoke for an hour-and-a-quarter and interacted well with the audience. People asked lots of questions and were particularly interested in my journey over the last five years. I was confident and loved what I was doing. The feedback afterwards was that I am amazing.

The thought of speaking in front of hundreds of people scares me, but I know I can do it. It's just a matter of feeling the fear and doing it anyway!

It brings me onto the £10 note metaphor

You have two £10 notes. One of them is pristine and new, whilst the other note has been used by many people; it has been torn in half and taped back together, scrunched up into a ball and thrown around, spat at and trodden on. After all the dishevelled £10 note has been through, it is still worth exactly the same as the pristine £10 note.

Whatever you have been through, you are still as important as everyone else in the world because life is priceless. You have loads of opportunities to do the things you love in life.

Thank you for reading *Stairs For Breakfast*. I hope I have inspired you.

If you have enjoyed this book, please give it a five-star rating on Amazon, along with an inspiring comment.

You can find a direct link to where this book is on Amazon by going to my website *www.stairsforbreakfast.com*.

You can also watch a short video of me and register to receive a free gift and updates on my journey.

I would like to inspire the world.

The Author

Patrick Souiljaert was born on the 21st November 1973, after having been deprived of oxygen for the first four minutes of his life. This caused his Cerebral Palsy which has been his constant companion ever since. This is a condition that makes dealing with the physical demands of life very difficult, but does not impair in any way the normal functions of the brain. In this respect Patrick has been blessed with more than his fair share of intelligence, insight and courage.

To that list we can now add the skill of writer and autobiographer. *Stairs For Breakfast* covers the period from November 1973 to September 2000. The sequel is planned for publication in Spring 2018.

Patrick has spent his life refusing to accept second best, compromise or to be labelled 'disabled'. He has insisted from his early years at school on being treated just like everyone else. This led him to an early career with a household corporate company, and a parallel career in radio where he worked with three local radio stations in Sussex as Producer. With his decision to take voluntary redundancy from his corporate job, Patrick embarked on a journey to pursue an ambition to make a £1 million. His interest in property investment was initially the preferred route, but this book may accelerate the journey. Over the last few years – in property investment and writing *Stairs For Breakfast* – Patrick has found his purpose and enjoyment in life by helping and inspiring others on his journey to reaching his full potential

Patrick lives in Sussex and was born to Belgian and English parents. He has a sister and a large collection of devoted friends.

Please could you help me to promote my book by giving it a five-star rating on Amazon, along with an inspiring comment. You can find a direct link to where this book is on Amazon by going to my website *www.stairsforbreakfast.com*.
I would like to inspire the world.
You can also watch a short video of me and sign up to my network. I'll email you a free gift and updates on my progress.

You can also buy my second book Screw It, I'll Take The Elevator!

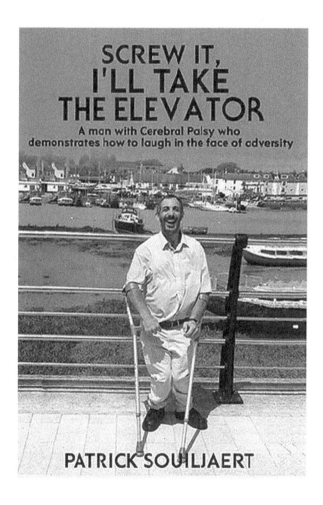